Bring Market Prices to Medicare

AEI STUDIES ON MEDICARE REFORM
Joseph Antos and Robert B. Helms
Series Editors

What ails Medicare is what ails health care in America. Medicare spending is growing substantially faster than we can afford, with potentially disastrous consequences for the federal budget. Worse, although the program is paying for more services, it is not necessarily providing better care for the elderly and the disabled. AEI's Studies on Medicare Reform is designed to examine the program's operation, consider alternative policy options, and develop a set of realistic proposals that could form the basis for reform legislation.

Bring Market Prices to Medicare

Essential Reform at a Time of Fiscal Crisis

Robert F. Coulam
Roger Feldman
Bryan E. Dowd

The AEI Press

Publisher for the American Enterprise Institute

WASHINGTON, D.C.

Distributed to the Trade by National Book Network, 15200 NBN Way, Blue Ridge Summit, PA 17214. To order call toll free 1-800-462-6420 or 1-717-794-3800. For all other inquiries please contact the AEI Press, 1150 Seventeenth Street, N.W., Washington, D.C. 20036 or call 1-800-862-5801.

Library of Congress Cataloging-in-Publication Data

Coulam, Robert F., 1948-
  Bring market prices to Medicare : essential reform at a time of fiscal crisis / Robert Coulam, Roger Feldman, and Bryan E. Dowd.
      p. ; cm.
  Includes bibliographical references and index.
  ISBN-13: 978-0-8447-4321-9
  ISBN-10: 0-8447-4321-6
  1. Medicare--Economic aspects. 2. Health care reform--United States.
I. Feldman, Roger D. II. Dowd, Bryan. III. Title.
  [DNLM: 1. Medicare--economics. 2. Competitive Medical
Plans—economics—United States. 3. Economic Competition—United
States. 4. Health Care Reform--United States. WT 31 C8543b 2009]
  RA412.3.C68 2009
  368.4'2600973—dc22

                                                              2009043596
13 12 11 10 09   1 2 3 4 5 6 7

Printed in the United States of America

Contents

List of Tables

Acknowledgments

The authors would like to thank the American Enterprise Institute for financial support to write this book, and also to thank Joseph Antos, Robert Berenson, Jeff Lemieux, Henry Olsen, Andrew Rettenmeier, and the Honorable Bill Thomas for their helpful comments.

Introduction

Medicare is the main government health insurance program for the elderly.[1] As anyone who follows the news is aware, the program faces critical financial difficulties. This book addresses one aspect of those difficulties: how the government determines its contributions to premiums for Medicare coverage. Current methods cost too much and fund more generous benefits for beneficiaries in some geographic areas than for beneficiaries in others. Here we propose a better method: competitive pricing.

Since the early years of the program, beneficiaries have had two options for receiving their Medicare coverage: through a public plan—the fee-for-service (FFS) Medicare plan, which enrolls about 80 percent of elderly beneficiaries—or through private health plans, mainly Medicare health maintenance organizations (HMOs). For decades, Medicare has determined its contributions to private plans' premiums based on costs of providing FFS coverage, with the precise method and its average generosity varying over time.

Government payments determined this way are inefficient, for reasons we will describe. We propose instead that Medicare move to a market-like arrangement, which we call "competitive pricing," to determine how much to pay FFS and private plans. (We generally ignore Medicare prescription drug coverage, which already uses a form of competitive pricing.)

If this book were written about any other health insurance program in the country, it would be greeted with a yawn. Competitive pricing is common—indeed, it is standard practice—throughout the health system, for large and small employers and for government health programs of all kinds, including Medicaid and the health programs of the U.S. Department of Defense and Department of Veterans Affairs. The application of competitive pricing to Medicare follows a set of simple premises:

- A basic Medicare benefit—the "entitlement"—is determined by Congress.

1

- The government's job is to buy the entitlement benefit package for all beneficiaries in the least expensive way possible, holding quality at a level that currently is acceptable and is improving over time.

- Competitive pricing is *by far* the most economical and efficient way for the government to accomplish that job.

- Our conclusion, given that the program faces a severe fiscal crisis, is that the government must adopt competitive pricing for Medicare.

The competitive pricing system we are proposing is no different from the system under which many beneficiaries have lived for decades while they were working. Its application to Medicare involves some technical challenges, but these have been solved many times by employers and other government programs and have been worked through in preparation for Medicare demonstrations.

Our proposal does involve one controversial premise that many do not accept: that Medicare should be an entitlement to a set of benefits, not to a particular way of financing or delivering those benefits. In the chapters that follow, we describe why that change in assumptions is essential to Medicare payment reform.

The urgency in our proposal for reform comes from the severity of the program's financial crisis. The *2009 Annual Report* of the Medicare trustees (U.S. Boards of Trustees 2009) warns that the Medicare hospital insurance trust fund will pay out more in benefits than it receives in revenues by 2017. Withdrawals from the trust fund that pays for physicians' services will grow substantially faster than the economy over time. These financial predictions make it imperative that Medicare find ways to reduce costs. As summarized by the U.S. Medicare Payment Advisory Commission (MedPAC):

[The] Medicare trustees and others warn of a serious mismatch between the benefits and payments the program currently provides and the financial resources available for the future. If Medicare benefits and payments systems remain as they are today, the trustees note that over time the program will require

major new sources of financing and impose a significant financial liability on taxpayers. Medicare beneficiaries will pay for rising expenditures through higher premiums and cost sharing.
Analysts across the political spectrum have raised concerns that
the current programs may become too heavy a fiscal burden and
squeeze the funding for other federal priorities. . . .

Delaying action would constrain the options for addressing
Medicare's problems. . . . As cost increases continue to outstrip
revenue and the retirement of the baby boom generation draws
closer, the time for phasing in major changes is growing shorter.
(U.S. Medicare Payment Advisory Commission 2009, xiii–xiv)

The problems MedPAC describes go well beyond payments to private
plans. But Medicare needs to address payment system reform now, when
substantial changes can be introduced more gently. Competitive pricing
is not the whole solution to Medicare's financial problems, but it can be
part of the solution. It should be established now to resolve the Medicare
payment problem for all health plans—public and private. *It is difficult
to imagine any other reform that could rationalize how Medicare pays public
and private plans, by bringing those payments closer to the cost of efficient
provision of the services Medicare covers.* The alternative to competitive pricing is a continuous political tug-of-war, resulting in fluctuations between
paying private plans too much or too little. Instead, we advocate establishing a level playing field with the same rules for both public and private
health plans.

To clarify this argument, it will be helpful first to provide some background on the Medicare program and the role and history of private plans
in Medicare.[2]

Background on the Medicare Program

Established in 1965, Medicare was initially intended to provide health
insurance to individuals ages sixty-five and older, regardless of income or
medical history. Medicare presently consists of four parts, each covering different benefits and offered under different funding and other arrangements.

- Part A, the hospital insurance (HI) program, covers inpatient hospital, skilled nursing, home health, and hospice care. It is funded through a tax on earnings paid by employers and workers.[3] In 2008, Part A benefit payments for FFS enrollees accounted for approximately 40 percent of Medicare benefit spending.

- Part B, the supplementary medical insurance (SMI) program, covers physician, outpatient, and preventive services, as well as certain home health services not covered under Part A. It is funded by general revenues and beneficiary premiums ($96.40 per month for most beneficiaries in 2009). Medicare beneficiaries who have higher annual incomes pay higher, income-related, monthly Part B premiums. In 2008, Part B services for FFS enrollees accounted for 27 percent of benefit spending.

- Part C, also known as the Medicare Advantage program, is of central concern in this book. Part C allows a beneficiary to enroll in a private health insurance plan, such as an HMO, preferred provider organization (PPO), or private fee-for-service (PFFS) plan. In the discussion that follows, we generally refer to these entities collectively as HMOs or private plans, except when the distinction among plan types matters for the discussion. These plans receive payments from Medicare to provide Medicare-covered Part A and B benefits, including hospital and physician services, and in most cases receive separate payments to cover prescription drug benefits as well. Part C is not separately financed—there is no separate fund, tax, or stream of government revenue earmarked for it. In 2008, government payments to Part C plans totaled 21 percent of Medicare benefit payments.

- Part D is the outpatient prescription drug benefit that was authorized by the Medicare Modernization Act of 2003 (MMA) and launched in 2006. Part D benefits are delivered through private plans that contract with Medicare. These may be either standalone prescription drug plans (PDPs) or Medicare Advantage prescription drug (MA-PD) plans. Part D plans are required to provide a standard benefit (or one that is equivalent) and may provide enhanced benefits. Individuals with modest incomes and assets are eligible for additional assistance with premiums and cost-sharing amounts. Part D is funded by general revenues, beneficiary premiums, and state payments, and in 2008 it accounted for 11 percent of benefit spending.

For beneficiaries enrolled in FFS for parts A and B, the government pays qualified providers a fee for each medically necessary service covered by the Medicare benefit (hence, the generally accurate label, "fee-for-service"). FFS enrollees pay the Part B premium, plus applicable copayments and deductibles set by Medicare for their care.

For beneficiaries enrolled in Part C, the government makes payments to health plans, not providers. The payments are in the form of a basic monthly payment per enrollee, risk-adjusted for enrollee characteristics and health conditions—a practice known as "risk contracting," because the government contracts with the private plan to take over the risk of health care spending by the plan's enrollees. Part C enrollees have to pay any additional premium (over the Part B amount) that the particular HMO charges, but copayments and deductibles typically are low or nonexistent in market areas where the government payment exceeds the plan's expenses.[4] The plans pay providers using their normal payment methods (such as capitation or discounted fees).

The History of Private Plans in Medicare

Medicare originally was modeled exclusively after fee-for-service health insurance offered by employers. Even by the early 1970s, however, costs were out of control. The Nixon administration determined that Medicare HMOs were an attractive remedy. In 1972, Congress added section 1876 to Title 18 of the Social Security Act, authorizing a new method of payment for HMOs. The law was a failure for a variety of reasons (Dowd, Feldman, and Christianson 1996; Williams 2005). Only one HMO elected to contract with Medicare until changes were made to the law in 1982, when Congress passed the Tax Equity and Fiscal Responsibility Act (TEFRA), which incorporated changes designed to encourage more plans to contract with Medicare. This statute marked the real beginning of Medicare risk contracting with HMOs. Enrollment in private health plans soared from less than one million in 1986 to over six million by early 1997, as managed care and the virtues of coordinated care dominated America's health-care landscape (Williams 2005).

In the early 1990s, research findings showed that private plans were overpaid due to inadequate adjustment for the health risks of their enrollees (Brown et al. 1993). In the mid-1990s, President Bill Clinton and the new Republican Congress worked together to balance the federal budget, in part, by reducing payments to private health plans in Medicare:

> In 1997, Congress and President Clinton agreed on a . . . framework for balancing the budget. The subsequent Balanced Budget Act (BBA) of 1997 reduced the rate of growth in Medicare spending by $112 billion for FY 1998 to FY 2002, making it the single largest contributor to balancing the budget. The Congressional Budget Office (CBO) projected that the bulk of that savings, $78.1 billion, would come from reducing payments to nearly all fee-for-service providers, and $21.8 billion from net reductions to private plans. (Williams 2005, 2)

The BBA created a new name for the private health plan program, Medicare+Choice (M+C), and established three new types of health plans to expand the range of consumer choice: preferred provider organizations (PPOs), private fee-for-service plans (PFFS), and provider-sponsored organizations (PSOs). Following the BBA reductions in plan payments, many plans withdrew from the Medicare market, reduced benefits, or increased cost-sharing and premiums. Congressional efforts to moderate the BBA effects on participation and enrollment, in the 1999 Medicare, Medicaid, and SCHIP Balanced Budget Refinement Act (BBRA) and the 2000 Medicare, Medicaid, and SCHIP Benefits Improvement and Protection Act (BIPA), were ineffective. Private plan participation and enrollment continued to drop. The majority of plans that remained in Medicare increased premiums and cost-sharing requirements, while reducing extra benefits.

In 2003, Congress enacted the Medicare Prescription Drug, Improvement, and Modernization Act (MMA). In addition to establishing Medicare Part D and other major reforms, the MMA made a substantial change in how Medicare contracted with health plans. It renamed the Medicare+Choice program the Medicare Advantage (MA) program and introduced a new plan type: the regional PPO. Regional PPOs were designed to improve beneficiaries' access to private plans by requiring PPOs to enter markets regionally, starting in 2006 (Pizer, Frakt, and Feldman 2007). The MMA also sought to increase plan participation by providing higher payments "intended to stabilize and expand the Medicare private plan market" (Williams 2005).

While there have been further legislative changes since MMA, no major changes have occurred in the types of health plans participating in Medicare. And the recent steps to encourage beneficiary enrollment in prepaid health plans have been successful, increasing enrollment from fewer than five million beneficiaries in prepaid plans of all types in 2003 to nearly ten million in 2008 (U.S. Medicare Payment Advisory Commission 2009).

Plan participation has mirrored this increase in enrollment, and the prepaid health plans on average have provided more generous benefits than were available to beneficiaries in FFS under the BBA. These increases in enrollment, participation, and benefits came at a price, however: In 2008, the Part C program on average cost 14 percent more per comparable beneficiary than the FFS program.

Throughout the history of private plans summarized above, a series of different goals are apparent:[5]

- *Cost control.* President Nixon and others viewed private health plans as more economical than FFS. They sought to introduce private plans as a way of controlling Medicare costs. In subsequent years, even as the private plans generally showed higher costs per beneficiary, the political support for them was still based on the assumption that they had the means and, with appropriate payment and risk adjustment, the incentives to provide cost control superior to that of the FFS plan.

- *Improvement in benefits and choice.* Private plans have the ability to offer more flexible formulations of the Part A and B benefits, as well as enhanced benefits and reduced premiums, within the requirement to offer equivalence to the statutory minimum benefit. This opportunity to move beyond "one size fits all," combined with the plans' ability to reduce costs relative to FFS

Medicare in some market areas, would provide consumers with more generous and diverse choices.[6]

- *Increased choice of plan types.* Many of the initiatives, including the BBA and the MMA, sought explicitly to introduce new types of plans, often in imitation of private commercial health insurance markets, as a means to give consumers more options.

- *Increase in plan participation and beneficiary enrollment.* Some initiatives, such as the original TEFRA statute and the MMA payment and other increases, have sought to increase plan participation and enrollment, typically in reaction to earlier declines.

These goals have often conflicted. Most important, aspirations to improve beneficiary enrollment, increase plan participation, and enhance benefits and choice have conflicted with the need to control costs. Indeed, something of a cycle has been happening between initiatives for cost control (in the mid-1990s leading to the BBA, and in 2008–9 as a new administration has taken office) and initiatives to expand enrollment, participation, benefits, and choice (notably, in 2003 in the MMA).

In this book, we do not argue for any particular level or balance between cost control on the one hand and increasing enrollment, participation, benefits, and choice on the other. We believe it would be prudent at a time of imminent financial crisis, however, to decide first what the appropriate Medicare care benefit should be, *and then determine the government contribution or payments needed to purchase that benefit most efficiently.* That concern leads us to focus on how the government sets its contribution to health plans and the incentives it creates for beneficiaries to select high-quality options that cost the government less. In the next section, we provide more detailed background on an issue noted in passing in the legislative history above: how the government contribution to private plans has been determined over time.

Payments to Private Health Plans

A central issue in this book is how the government determines what to pay health plans in Part C. From its first efforts to contract with private health plans, Medicare has struggled to find a satisfactory method to calculate payments. It has used three identifiable approaches.

The first was based on simple risk adjustments to a capitation rate set at 95 percent of the average cost of caring for beneficiaries in FFS Medicare in each county. This method, which became the "adjusted average percapita cost" (AAPCC) system, did not track HMO costs very well. HMOs in some market areas offered enhanced benefits, often including outpatient prescription drug coverage, without any additional premium. Plans in other areas charged substantial premiums for coverage that differed little from the basic entitlement. Meanwhile, in many areas (especially rural areas), no private health plans were available to Medicare beneficiaries. By the mid-1990s, few independent observers had anything good to say about the AAPCC, but it provided generous payments in enough areas to increase HMO ("Medicare+Choice") enrollment to 17 percent of all elderly beneficiaries in 1999 (U.S. Department of Health and Human Services, Centers for Medicare and Medicaid Services 1999).

In response to the expense and uneven generosity of the AAPCC, Congress adopted a new payment method in the 1997 BBA legislation. The BBA and its refinements altered the direct link between FFS costs and payments. The generosity of payments in relation to plan costs in high-payment areas was moderated. Medicare saved money compared with the AAPCC method, but the reductions in reimbursement compared with former methods led to substantial declines in plan participation and Medicare enrollment. Williams notes:

> When Congress enacted the BBA in 1997, it assumed that the private health plan market would continue growing. However, an industry-wide shift in strategies from growing enrollment and market share toward restoring profitability, combined with rising health care costs and Medicare reductions in plan payments, produced a different outcome. Plans withdrew from the Medicare market, reduced benefits, or increased cost-sharing and premiums. (Williams 2005, 3)

The number of participating plans declined from 346 in 1998 to 157 in 2002 (U.S. Medicare Payment Advisory Commission 2004), and Medicare+Choice enrollment declined to 12 percent of beneficiaries by December

2003 (U.S. Department of Health and Human Services, Centers for Medicare and Medicaid Services 2003).

In 1999 and 2000, Congress began to step back from more stringent BBA methods. In 2003, the MMA instituted a nominal bidding system for Medicare Advantage plans in which the government set a so-called benchmark price, based on a series of rules that increased plan payments. According to MedPAC:

> The benchmark is a bidding target under the bidding system. . . . The local MA benchmarks come from the county-level payment rates used to pay MA plans before 2006. Those payment rates were at least as high as per capita fee-for-service (FFS) Medicare spending in each county. Some counties had rates significantly higher than FFS because of specific statutory changes. (U.S. Medicare Payment Advisory Commission 2007, 62)

The report further explains:

> [For] bids below the benchmark, the law requires that 75 percent of the difference (referred to as the rebate) be used to fund extra benefits for enrollees. The program keeps the remaining 25 percent in the Medicare trust funds. (Ibid., 61)

MA plans also were allowed to use their overpayment to buy down the Part B premium. Although the MMA method is a bidding system in form, the level of plan payments is influenced strongly by the administratively set benchmark price, which is not affected by plan bids. MA plans know the benchmark prior to submitting their bids. The 25 percent tax on low bids, like all taxes, discourages the taxed activity—in this case, the provision of supplementary benefits and premium rebates. Following passage of the MMA, Medicare Advantage enrollment reached a low of 12.1 percent of beneficiaries in 2004 before increasing to 19.5 percent in 2007 (U.S. Boards of Trustees 2008).

In current policy discussions, the generosity of MA payment methods has—predictably, one might say—given rise to proposals urging that the pendulum swing back to less generous payments. In 2008, MedPAC proposed to pay all plans at the level of fee-for-service costs (U.S. Medicare Payment

Advisory Commission 2008a). MedPAC's proposal would reduce overpayments to private plans, but it would exacerbate current geographic disparities in government-financed benefits—restoring them to pre-1997 BBA levels—and it would not allow the government to save money in areas where private plans can provide entitlement benefits more efficiently than FFS Medicare.

There are many other proposals in addition to MedPAC's, all of which would reduce payment to private plans. Robert Berenson, of the Urban Institute, argued for payments based on adjustments to FFS costs (Berenson 2008). More recently, the Obama administration announced technical changes in the calculation of the 2010 base payment rates for private health plans, which will reduce benchmark payments by almost 5 percent, compared with previous methods (U.S. Department of Health and Human Services, Centers for Medicare and Medicaid Services 2009; Fuhrmans and Zhang 2009). The administration also proposed a new competitive pricing system for determining private health plans' rates. The bidding system would only involve Medicare Advantage plans—that is, FFS would be excluded from the bidding. Plans in each geographic area would submit bids on a standard benefit. An important difference between the Obama proposal and the MedPAC proposal is that in the Obama proposal, MA plans would not know the "benchmark" government payment prior to submitting their bids. The benchmark would be set at the average of the plan bids. Plans whose bids exceeded that benchmark would have to charge beneficiaries a premium for the difference. Plans bidding under that amount would be permitted to offer enhancements, such as improved benefits or reduced premiums.

The Obama proposal closely resembles the design of the failed competitive pricing demonstrations of the mid- to late 1990s. It would be an improvement over the current payment system and the MedPAC and Berenson proposals because the plans would be bidding against an unknown benchmark—a design that is likely to produce lower bids. FFS Medicare still would be protected from competition with private plans, however—a feature that not only increases the cost of the program, but also opens the Obama administration to the criticism that the federal government is incapable of administering a level playing field and instead will favor its own FFS plan in a competitive bidding system. Against all these proposals, the private health plan industry argues in favor of continuing the current policy and proposes to explore other ways to achieve Medicare savings.

In this book, we urge a different approach: competitive pricing for all health plans, including FFS Medicare as well as private plans, based on bids for a basic entitlement benefit package submitted by those plans for each area they serve.[7] The entitlement could remain as it is today, or it could be defined differently by Congress. The government's contribution to premiums would be equal to the lowest bid from any plan or—more for political than economic reasons—perhaps some other amount, such as the mean or median bid. Having determined the government's contribution to the basic benefit package, all plans would be free to sell additional supplementary coverage at whatever price the market would bear.

Competitive pricing has a substantial history in Medicare. In the second half of the 1990s, at the time the AAPCC was being replaced by the BBA method, the Centers for Medicare and Medicaid Services (CMS) mounted efforts to implement a demonstration of competitive pricing for HMOs. (FFS was excluded, as in the Obama administration's current proposal.) In four different attempts, the demonstration was blocked because it would have disrupted politically influential groups of beneficiaries and health plans. The demonstration efforts ended as the BBA continued to be implemented with legislative refinements.

At the time the MMA was being debated, competitive pricing for Medicare health plans was again considered by a significant group of congressional Republicans. Pressures to introduce competitive pricing were deflected by the standard legislative device of requiring a demonstration, but making sure that it was many years off. Few took this comparative cost adjustment (CCA) demonstration seriously when the MMA created it.[8] But time passes, and the demonstration is now scheduled to take place in 2010.[9] Serious opposition has begun to mobilize, and there are signs the demonstration may be canceled (amendments to do so have been introduced in Congress, though not yet passed).

Our proposal is based on many of the same criticisms of current payment policy offered by MedPAC, Berenson, and the Obama administration. Most important, we agree that current payments to Medicare Advantage plans are too high, and the magnitude of the difference (especially for plans with weak claims to improved quality—notably PFFS plans) is unsupportable at a time when the program faces a substantial financial crisis. Where we part ways with other analysts is our simple and symmetrical observation that in some market areas, payments to FFS Medicare are too high, and the magnitude of that difference is also unsupportable at a time when the program faces a substantial financial crisis.

We disagree with MedPAC and Berenson on the answer to a deceptively simple question: How should the government's contribution to Medicare premiums (sometimes referred to as the "benchmark") be set? MedPAC's proposal assumes payments to plans can get no closer to the plans' true costs than whatever the standardized local FFS costs happen to be. Berenson proposes adjusting private plans' payments under the MedPAC regime to push them closer to plans' costs, leaving FFS untouched. We propose a benchmark that is more reliably close to the cost of purchasing services from the most efficient plan in each local market. MedPAC and Berenson envision competition among private plans over benefits, given some agreement on a more economical price than current policy allows. Our proposal goes further and envisions competition among *all* plans over the most economical price for an agreed-upon set of entitlement benefits.

We also disagree with the Obama administration on some essential points of the bidding system it proposes. For example, as will be discussed below, the savings from competitive pricing are substantially reduced by setting the benchmark at the average bid, rather than the lowest qualified bid. We see no reason to subsidize less efficient plans. More fundamentally, we disagree with the exclusion of FFS from the bidding process. We expect that in some market areas FFS Medicare would be the low bidder, while in others a private plan would submit the lowest bid. If private health plans are more economical than FFS in a particular geographic area, have sufficient capacity, and meet appropriate quality standards, why should the government pay more? The government contribution should encourage beneficiaries to use more economical alternatives—private plans when they are more economical, FFS when it is. For those who immediately imagine vast beneficiary disruption from such an approach, we urge reserving judgment until they have read further: FFS would be the low bidder in geographic areas where 15 percent of all beneficiaries live; otherwise, private plans would be the low bidders. The differences would be less than 10 percent in most areas, however, and transition rules to buffer beneficiaries from any abrupt change would be easy to devise.

Finally, our proposal would remove the 25 percent tax on low bids. Under the current system, low bids are not entirely desirable from the government's perspective because most of the benefits (75 percent) accrue to beneficiaries, resulting in higher costs to taxpayers and increased fiscal pressure on the Medicare program. In that distorted environment, a tax on low bids might make some sense. Under our proposal, however, the savings from lower bids for the entitlement benefit package would accrue to the government. Taxpayers and beneficiaries would benefit from lower program costs and an extended fiscal life of the program. In that environment, we can think of no reason to tax low bids.

At a time when Medicare faces enormous fiscal problems, the program must stop overpaying for entitlement benefits and paying for benefits that are not part of the entitlement. Those who say a competitive pricing system that includes FFS Medicare must wait until FFS Medicare becomes more efficient have it backwards. The best way to ensure improvement in FFS Medicare is to subject it, not just MA plans, to the competitive pressure of the marketplace. Delay in these changes—"muddling through"—may be an expedient reaction to political pressures of the day, but in the long run it will threaten greater disruption to beneficiaries and less careful accommodation to beneficiary, health plan, and provider expectations. It is time to bring market prices to Medicare!

Outline of the Book

The outline of our book is as follows. Before discussing how to pay health plans in Medicare, we want to be sure that Medicare should offer beneficiaries both a private plan option and a government plan. Therefore, in chapter 1, we outline the purposes of Medicare as we see them, and we argue that they are best accomplished by a mixed public and private system, because the public plan and private plans both have advantages and disadvantages, in areas we will clearly spell out.

Once agreed that both types of plans should be offered, the question becomes one of designing an efficient and fair payment system. As indicated above, our choice is competitive pricing, specifically, a system that uses plans' bids—for example, their estimated cost of caring for their enrollees in some geographic area, such as a county—to set the government premium contribution for both private plans and FFS Medicare in that geographic area. The "bid" submitted by FFS Medicare would be the average cost of caring for a standardized beneficiary in FFS Medicare in the geographic area.

Chapter 2 explains why competitive pricing is better than the four options currently being considered: the current MA payment system, MedPAC's proposal for setting MA payments equal to the FFS level, Berenson's proposal to adjust MA payments using MA cost reports and other data, and the Obama administration's proposal to introduce a form of competitive pricing. Because MedPAC's proposal amounts to a return to the AAPCC, we spend much of chapter 2 explaining why the AAPCC had no defenders when it was used—a result that, we will argue, would be the fate of a return to pricing at FFS levels.

Despite its conceptual and administrative simplicity, competitive pricing entails a number of technical issues, which we discuss in chapter 3. The chapter begins with an explanation of the current payment arrangements for three types of MA plans—local coordinated-care plans, regional preferred provider organizations, and private fee-for-service plans. Since these arrangements involve a form of bidding, albeit against known benchmarks that do not depend on plans' bids, we ask whether plans' bids in the *current* "bidding" system reflect their costs. The answer to this question will affect our estimate of the savings from competitive pricing in the following chapter.

The short answer is a qualified "Yes," but the qualifications are important. Exclusion of FFS Medicare from the current system—which implies that MA plans can give premium rebates but cannot force FFS to charge more than the Part B premium—may weaken MA plans' motivation to submit low bids. In addition, bidding against a known benchmark, as in the current system, is likely to create less competitive pressure on plans than bidding against an unknown benchmark determined from the plans' bids themselves.

In the second part of chapter 3, we compare different ways of setting the government premium contribution. We suggest that, despite the theoretical appeal of some alternatives, our proposal for setting it equal to the lowest bid would save more money for Medicare than setting it equal to the second-lowest bid. (All of our discussion about bids rests on the assumption that they have been adjusted for the health risk of the plan's enrollees.) We discuss problems that may arise when the contribution is based on the lowest bid, but recommend that the government be wary of rejecting any bids just because they seem "unreasonably" low.

Chapter 4 presents estimates of the savings from competitive pricing. We review past estimates of the savings from the Medicare HMO program and from competitive pricing models that rely on bids from HMOs as well as FFS Medicare to set the government payment rate. Next, we calculate the likely savings from MedPAC's proposal (U.S. Medicare Advisory Commission 2007a; U.S. House of Representatives, Committee on the Budget 2007) for "leveling the playing field" by paying all plans at the level of FFS cost, and we compare these to estimates of the savings from competitive pricing. MedPAC's proposal would save only a very small amount of money, as would average-bid models that use both FFS's and HMOs' bids to create a single weighted-average bid and MA-only models that use the average of the bids (the Obama proposal). Competitive pricing models that use the lower of the average HMO bid or the FFS bid to set the payment rate for all plans would save more money. The most effective payment system in terms of savings would use the lowest bid from any qualified health plan (FFS or HMO) to set the payment rate for all Medicare plans.

We recognize that our proposal would result in disruption for some beneficiaries, in terms of potentially substantial increases in the cost of their health plans. In chapter 4 we explain approximately how much disruption would occur, and which beneficiaries would be most affected. The identification of these beneficiaries is the first step in thinking about special efforts to minimize short-term disruption and enable beneficiaries to make satisfactory longer-term adjustments.

If FFS Medicare is to be part of the "mix" of competitive pricing, it is reasonable to ask whether FFS should be allowed greater flexibility (that is, to act more like an MA plan). Chapter 5 discusses several ways to accomplish that, such as allowing FFS to make investments in administrative improvements and offering an alternative plan.

The political opposition that has blocked competitive pricing in the past raises an important caution. Chapter 6 faces the fact that all efforts to establish competitive pricing in Medicare have failed, despite several cases in which bidding resulted in substantial savings without adverse effects on quality. We attribute the failure of these nominally successful past efforts to opposition from health plans and providers, and fears of *potential* harm to beneficiaries from competitive pricing. We suggest some modest steps to overcome such opposition, although we recognize that the political feasibility of competitive pricing is not merely a matter of strategy or tactics. It is likely to require, most importantly, a change in the political environment—a realization that Medicare's uneconomical payment methods cannot be sustained.

Overall, we argue that the best way to address opposition to needed reforms is not to minimize the extent of the reform, but rather to recognize reasonable beneficiary needs and expectations by making a slow transition to this longer-term goal (at least for all beneficiaries who face disruption), allowing adjustments in enrollment choices and expectations. We should tell current *and future* beneficiaries *now* that this is where the program is headed and why, rather than pretending that more incremental reforms can accomplish similar results. We expect that future beneficiaries will find a competitive pricing system in Medicare less disruptive than current beneficiaries. Many future beneficiaries will have spent their working lives choosing health plans in a competitive pricing environment.

Given our view that competitive pricing is the most desirable payment option, it would seem logical to have a demonstration of this concept. In chapter 7, however, we argue that this is not necessary, and that we should implement competitive pricing nationally without first demonstrating it, for two reasons. First, we already know almost everything that could be learned from a demonstration. Competitive pricing is feasible, and the CMS has shown that it is quite capable of administering such a system. Competitive pricing is an administratively straightforward extension of current payment policy, as it builds naturally on the current MMA system of quasi-bids from health plans. Employers offering multiple health plans to their employees have used various forms of competitive pricing for decades, and those that set a level-dollar contribution to the premiums of all health plans, as opposed to a level percentage contribution or other approach, have enjoyed the lowest premiums. We also know from the experiences of both the private commercial insurance sector and the demonstrations of competitive pricing in Medicare in the 1990s that competition works—in the case of Medicare, producing bids in one high-payment market area that were substantially lower than MA payment levels.

Second, recent history suggests, paradoxically, that demonstrations of major reforms that affect only a subset of Medicare beneficiaries are not politically viable, whereas significant reforms that affect all beneficiaries have been successfully implemented through program-wide changes. To reduce political opposition, we recommend moving toward competitive pricing gradually so that beneficiaries, health plans, and providers have time to adapt.

Finally, in the conclusion, we summarize our argument and offer some closing remarks.

Competitive pricing for all Medicare health plans will not solve Medicare's fiscal problems; among other reasons, competitive pricing has no important effect on certain secular increases in health-care costs, or on the dramatic increase in the size of the beneficiary population. None of the other health plan payment reforms will affect those other sources of cost either. Competitive pricing can, however,

- save money for the Medicare program;

- remove the subsidies that distort the government's decisions regarding the Medicare entitlement benefit package;

- end political bickering over administratively determined MA payments; and

- stabilize payment policy for MA plans. Competitive prices provide the obvious equilibrium for payment policy between the systematic overpayments of current policy and the arbitrary over- and underpayments of FFS levels and methods like the BBA.

Supporters of the Medicare program often note its popularity with current beneficiaries. Unfortunately, that support is tied directly to the program's fiscal mismanagement. Any health plan, public or private, would likely be equally popular with beneficiaries if they paid only a fraction of the cost of coverage.

Medicare's critics are concerned that we are passing the program's costs on to our children. As irresponsible as that sounds, it actually would be an improvement over the current situation. The Medicare program faces a $32.9 trillion unfunded deficit over the next seventy-five years. That is not the cost of the program, nor is it the portion of the cost that we are passing on to our children. It is the part of the cost for which no one is even bothering to make up a funding story.

Saving the Medicare program is likely to involve a combination of higher premiums, higher taxes, and reduced program costs, achieved through a variety of methods that will involve major concessions on the part of beneficiaries, particularly beneficiaries in areas of the country with high health-care spending per capita. The sooner we begin making the required changes, the less painful they will be, and the more time we can give future beneficiaries to prepare for them. The alternative is the intentional, orchestrated crises that are the foundation of poor public policy.

1

The Purposes of Medicare

Obviously, competitive pricing would require a statutory change in how FFS Medicare is offered to beneficiaries, since it would require beneficiaries to pay more than the Part B premium to enroll in FFS in those areas where FFS is more expensive than at least one qualified local MA plan. For example, if average risk-adjusted costs in a given county for the entitlement benefit package in FFS Medicare were $750 per beneficiary per month, and the lowest risk-adjusted bid by an MA plan were $700 per beneficiary per month, beneficiaries in that county who wished to enroll in FFS Medicare would have to pay an additional $50 per month, over and above their Part B premium. They could, however, avoid the additional charge by joining the lowest-cost MA plan.

Opponents of competitive pricing refer to this result as "herding," or forcing beneficiaries into MA plans. That is a misnomer, and we have no desire to herd or force any beneficiary into any health plan. We do, however, want beneficiaries *to face the true price differentials between more efficient health plans and less efficient health plans*, and to make health plan choices with those differences in mind, first, because beneficiaries then will pick plans that provide the best value for the money and, second, because doing so gives all health plans a strong incentive to become more efficient. We also point out that structuring subsidies so that beneficiaries can enroll in FFS Medicare for the Part B premium regardless of FFS Medicare's true cost relative to MA plans can be viewed as herding or forcing beneficiaries into FFS Medicare, and that policy is equally objectionable.

Any requirement that beneficiaries pay more than the applicable Part B premium to enroll in FFS would require changes in Medicare's governing statutes and in beneficiary expectations about what FFS is. The key question is whether such changes would be so contradictory to the purposes of the Medicare program that they should not be considered—thus making competitive pricing as we have defined it impossible.

The best place to begin this discussion is to ask, "What are the purposes of the Medicare program?" While there is room for argument, we believe the program embodies five major purposes:

- To protect currently eligible beneficiaries against random varia- tion in health-care spending—the standard purpose of health insurance;

- to insure against some of the health-care costs associated with disability and end-stage renal disease (ESRD);

- to guarantee that beneficiaries who become eligible for Medicare will never have their coverage terminated for any reason other than failure to pay their Part B, C, and D premiums;

- to guarantee that beneficiaries are protected against premium increases (for some fixed, minimum level of coverage) due to changes in their health status; and

- to provide a safety net that protects beneficiaries from outliving their assets—accomplished by requiring no beneficiary pre- mium for Part A and substantial premium subsidies for Parts B, C, and D, as well as by providing dual eligibility for Medicare and Medicaid.

Our first observation is that all of these purposes could be fulfilled by either a public plan (FFS) or private plans. Thus, at least in terms of these purposes, it is not essential that FFS Medicare be available everywhere for the Part B premium alone if at least one qualified MA plan is available for a lower price than FFS Medicare.

Our second observation is that the purposes of the Medicare program are reflected, legislatively, in the *entitlement benefit package*—the package of benefits that is available to Medicare beneficiaries by law in all parts of the United States. Curiously, in an era of free prescription drugs, free trans- portation to medical facilities, and health club memberships for beneficiar- ies in areas of high MA payments, we have found it necessary to remind even seasoned policy analysts that there actually is a Medicare entitlement benefit package that does not include these services. If Congress considered coverage of prescription drugs, or health club memberships, or access to any provider willing to accept the FFS Medicare fee schedule regardless of geographic location, to be essential to carrying out the purposes of the Medicare program, then those benefits and coverage levels would be required of every Medicare health plan, including FFS Medicare and private health plans.

Third, both the public FFS Medicare plan and some private plans cover services beyond the entitlement benefit package. Coverage of these additional, or "supplementary," benefits will result in higher costs for the plan that provides them. Obviously, if the cost of such a plan is used to set the government's contribution to premiums for all beneficiaries, then the Medicare budget will reflect the cost of those supplementary features that are not part of the Medicare entitlement. For example, MedPAC has proposed that Medicare return to the pre-1998 practice of setting its contribution to health plan premiums at the level of average FFS spending in each county. There are two important features that are required only of FFS Medicare and not of private plans: open access to all participating providers without a referral and equal coverage of all providers regardless of their locations— a feature we refer to as a "national service area." These features are not required of all health plans in Medicare, and thus we conclude that Congress does not consider them essential to carrying out the purposes of the Medicare program. They unquestionably increase the cost of FFS Medicare, however, and basing the government's contribution to premiums for all beneficiaries on the cost of a plan that includes those benefits—that is, FFS Medicare—artificially inflates the cost of the Medicare program.

Reasons to Offer a Public Plan and Private Plans

Our review of the purposes of the Medicare program suggests that those purposes might be accomplished with either a public plan or private health plans. We think, however, they are best accomplished by a mixed public and private system, because the public plan and private plans both have advantages and disadvantages. Here we express the advantages and disadvantages of private health plans in Medicare *relative* to the public plan, and vice versa. Thus, each advantage of one plan type is mirrored by a disadvantage of the other.[1] We organize the advantages and disadvantages into three areas: areas where FFS Medicare has advantages over private plans; areas where private plans have advantages over FFS Medicare; and areas where the evidence is mixed.

Areas Where FFS Medicare Has Advantages. FFS Medicare has three notable advantages over private plans.

Universal geographic availability: An entitlement to which some eligible beneficiaries living in the United States did not have any access would be unacceptable. FFS Medicare (the public plan) has a history of offering insurance coverage to all beneficiaries, nationwide. Only since 2006 have private health plans been available nationwide (U.S. Senate, Committee on Finance 2008).[2] Because FFS has national availability, beneficiaries know that regardless of where they live in the United States, they will have access to a health plan that offers the entitlement benefit package.[3]

Geographic stability of out-of-pocket premiums: Medicare beneficiaries pay an out-of-pocket premium for Part B that is uniform nationwide and thus more geographically stable than private plan premiums in Medicare that vary from one geographic area to another, in part because the mix of private plans and the government's premium contribution varies from one area to another. Whether the geographic uniformity of the Part B premium is desirable depends on the explanation for dramatic variations in average county-level FFS spending. For example, if the variation is due purely to the inefficient provision of health-care services, why should beneficiaries in low-cost areas and (all) taxpayers subsidize that activity?

Economies of scale: FFS Medicare is the largest health plan in the United States. If health plans operate with substantial economies of scale— primarily in processing claims—then FFS Medicare should be able to exploit them. Economies of scale in health plans appear to be quite limited, however. Wholey and others (1996) found that economies of scale in Medicare health plans are exhausted at approximately 12,000 enrollees—below the enrollment of most private plans, and far below the 35 million beneficiaries in FFS Medicare.

Areas Where Private Plans Have Advantages. Private plans have advantages in at least six areas.

Access to care. To qualify for participation in Medicare, private health plans must have provider networks that guarantee a minimal level of access to care for Medicare beneficiaries. FFS Medicare guarantees only to cover the cost of participating health-care providers. Although periodic surveys of access to care are conducted by various agencies, the statutory FFS Medicare entitlement does not guarantee that any providers within a reasonable distance of a beneficiary's place of residence will accept Medicare patients.

Coordination of coverage and services. The artificial division of Medicare into Part A, Part B, and Part D has made it difficult to institute payment reforms—for instance, bundling of inpatient and outpatient services—that would encourage greater efficiency in the delivery of care. MA plans are paid a capitation rate that is a composite of calculated Part A and Part B rates, but the MA plan is free to divide the revenue among services and pay providers in any way it sees fit. FFS Medicare is prohibited from offering outpatient drug coverage and thus must rely on private insurers to cover both supplementary services (beyond the entitlement) and outpatient drugs—reducing opportunities to use the payment system to encourage coordination of care.

Flexibility in cost-sharing. Private Medicare plans are held to a standard of actuarial equivalence in their benefit designs—for example, they are able to substitute copayments for coinsurance and deductibles—and thus have greater freedom to experiment with consumer cost-sharing designs than FFS Medicare.

Disease management and care delivery. Whereas private plans have engaged in various types of care management for years (Welch 2002), FFS Medicare has only recently begun testing disease-management programs, and the results have been disappointing (Abelson 2008). Although MA plans are subject to the same coverage requirements as FFS Medicare, they can exercise greater control over the actual use of disease-management technology. The CMS currently lacks statutory authority to engage in disease management except in the context of demonstration projects.

Product diversity. Private Medicare plans can offer a variety of products with different benefits, provider networks, and other dimensions that might be important to consumers, whereas FFS Medicare offers only a standard entitlement benefit package, relying on private supplementary ("Medigap") insurers to offer additional levels of coverage at varying prices.

Incentives and freedom to pursue efficient purchasing strategies. Private plans, like all private producers, must balance the desires of their customers (enrollees) against the desires of their suppliers (health care providers). They have, however, a strong incentive to pursue efficient production of health care for their enrollees while maintaining consumer satisfaction. The penalty for failure is clear—reduced enrollment. The government's incentive to pursue the same types of efficiency is less clear. Even when the government is motivated to pursue efficiency, a large public plan may face greater barriers than smaller private plans. Purchasing decisions of any health plan that affect a large segment of the market can become politicized and subject to review by the legislature and the courts. If the plan is a federal government plan, it is likely that Congress will micromanage it.

As noted earlier, congressional management of FFS Medicare is uneven, but in some areas it is intense, including the area of setting physician fees. Members of Congress have expressed some frustration over the level of micromanagement they have taken on. Senate Finance Committee chair Max Baucus (D-Montana) recently remarked, "As a member of Congress, I sometimes wonder if we're competent to answer some of the questions we're called upon to [answer]." He added, "For example, how in the world am I supposed to know what the proper reimbursement rate should be for a certain procedure?" (KaiserNetwork.org 2008). Despite the occasional recognition of its limitations, however, Congress appears reluctant to delegate politically useful tasks to a more autonomous entity. As a result, it is subject to intense lobbying by health plans, providers, and others seeking increases in their payment rates.

Private plans currently are able to negotiate payment rates with their participating providers free of congressional oversight. They also are able to exclude providers from their networks purely on the basis of price, whereas the CMS must contract with all willing providers who meet basic participation criteria and are willing to accept FFS payment rates.

The CMS has attempted to purchase services such as durable medical equipment and clinical laboratory services through a competitive bidding process, but those efforts have been uniformly blocked by the courts and especially by Congress, even when Congress had mandated demonstrations of competitive purchasing. This remarkable history of obstruction—of keeping FFS from becoming a prudent purchaser of services—is documented in chapter 6. Congress may have allowed greater latitude to private plans in their provider-contracting practices, however, in part because the plans represent a relatively small share of the Medicare market. If their market share increases significantly, Congress may well increase its meddling in private plans' contracting practices.

Areas Where Evidence Is Mixed. In three areas the evidence is mixed, favoring neither public nor private plans, on balance.

Quality of care. Extensive reviews of the literature by Miller and Luft (1997, 2002) found that the quality of care in HMOs and FFS health plans was roughly equivalent. Much of that literature was based on the Medicare program. FFS Medicare was found to have a slight advantage in chronic care, while HMOs had a slight advantage in preventive care.

An important distinction between FFS Medicare and private Medicare plans is that private plans are required to report extensive information on quality of care under the Healthcare Effectiveness Data and Information Set (HEDIS) system[4] to the CMS, which then is publicly reported. FFS Medicare is exempt from HEDIS reporting requirements.

Administrative cost. Advocates of FFS Medicare frequently cite its low administrative cost—between 2 and 5 percent of the program's total budget (U.S. Congressional Budget Office 2006; U.S. Department of Health and Human Services, Centers for Medicare and Medicaid Services 2008; Mathews 2006) compared with the CMS's estimate of 11–13 percent of total premiums for private plans (U.S. Department of Health and Human Services, Centers for Medicare and Medicaid Services 2008). A point often lost in these discussions, however, is that the optimal level of expenditure on administration is not likely to be the minimal level. Any health plan could minimize its expenditures on administrative costs simply by paying every claim that is submitted, with no scrutiny whatsoever. The likely result would be rampant fraud and abuse. Minimally, we would expect an efficient health plan to be willing to spend a dollar on administration if doing so saved more than a dollar. Furthermore, we would expect an efficient health plan acting as a responsible agent for its enrollees to spend an additional dollar on administration even if there were no savings, as long as the expenditure resulted in an improvement in service for which enrollees were willing to pay at least a dollar. For example, a health plan might add more staff to its telephone help-lines to reduce waiting times if enrollees were willing to pay the cost of those additional staff.

The CMS and its contractors encounter the difficulty that administrative expenses can be paid only from a fund earmarked by Congress for administration, not from the funds that pay for beneficiaries' health expenses (Berenson and Dowd 2008). Thus, the CMS may be constrained from additional investment on administration, even when such investment would be cost-saving. Private plans face no such constraint.

Health plan pricing power. In markets with little competition, providers can reduce the supply of their services and drive up prices. Because FFS Medicare is the dominant buyer of a wide variety of health-care services and thus has considerable market buying power, it is able to counter that effect. FFS prices tend to be lower than those paid by commercial insurers and may be closer to competitive prices in markets with concentrated provider pricing power. This situation, referred to as "bilateral monopoly," can be an improvement over unopposed monopoly pricing power on the part of providers, but it is not better than the competitive pricing outcome that, in principle, would result from more aggressive enforcement of antitrust laws.

Moreover, FFS Medicare's pricing power has two disadvantages. First, it prevents FFS Medicare from responding to legitimate local variation in supply and demand conditions. Second, pricing power can be inefficient when it results in "monopsony" pricing in a previously competitive market for health-care services. When one buyer (FFS Medicare) controls the market-wide demand for providers' services, and that buyer wants to purchase more services, it must increase its payments to all providers in the market. As a result, the buyer tends to purchase fewer services, resulting in an inefficiently low level of output.

A related disadvantage of FFS Medicare's pricing power is that the program is large enough to affect the supply of services to the commercially insured and Medicaid populations. Access to providers is important, but should FFS Medicare set its fees high enough to eliminate all vestiges of access problems for its beneficiaries? When Medicare raises its fees to guarantee access for its beneficiaries, providers have less incentive to see commercially insured patients and thus are less willing to quote lower prices to commercial insurers. The result is an increase in commercial insurance premiums and higher rates of uninsurance. In the past, Medicare has conducted surveys of providers' willingness to see new FFS Medicare patients. To our knowledge, no one is monitoring the impact of Medicare fees on access to care in non-Medicare populations.

The Political Disadvantage of a Mixed-Plan System

Although we believe a system of private and public plans is superior to one limited to either type of plan, a mixed public and private system has an important political disadvantage: Congress micromanages the Medicare program. This micromanagement extends to policies that govern the participation of private plans in the Medicare program, and it permeates the management of traditional FFS Medicare. The political problem is that Congress is not of one mind regarding the participation of private health plans in Medicare. Some members would prefer to have only private plans in the Medicare program, while others apparently would prefer to have none. These polar views are brought to bear on the vast array of Medicare-related management decisions that Congress makes—each faction using each decision to try to move the program in its preferred direction.

The combatants in this ideological struggle hold different views of such fundamental concerns as

- the proper role of government;
- the ability of competition to discipline the price and quality of products in the market;

- the ability of and incentives for government employees to produce the combination of price, quality, and quantity of benefits that maximizes the welfare of current and future beneficiaries; and

- the promotion of "social solidarity" through enrolling all beneficiaries in one plan.

In the context of these ideological disputes, overarching issues like the long-run fiscal health of the program often are overlooked or treated as additional battlegrounds, thus threatening its very existence.

Unfortunately, this problem has no easy answer. One solution would be to satisfy one faction or the other by discarding either private health plans or FFS Medicare, but that is not going to happen, for the same reason the ideological struggles continue: Congress is not of one mind. Our view is that either approach would be undesirable as well as unrealistic.

Another solution proposed by some would be to turn administration of the program over to a different entity than Congress. But the CMS is such an agency. If members of Congress were inclined to let another agency take on the administration of the Medicare program, they could allow the CMS to do that now.

The record on Congress's ability to delegate responsibility to the CMS is mixed. The Medicare Modernization Act of 2003 gave the CMS a great deal of discretion to design and implement the Part D program, to which, in our opinion, the CMS responded very well. The production, testing, and installation of the consumer information system that supports the choice of Part D plans (including drug-specific, out-of-pocket cost comparisons for multiple plans and locations of their participating pharmacies) over an eighteen-month period ranks as one of the most impressive technological achievements in the history of consumer health-care information systems. On the other hand, as will be discussed in chapter 6, Congress has blocked (often after mandating) the CMS's efforts to purchase durable medical equipment through competitive bidding and even to *demonstrate* competitive bidding for clinical lab services and MA plan payment (Dowd, Coulam, and Feldman 2000).

It seems unlikely that Congress will be willing to reduce its hands-on management of the Medicare program. Thus, our working assumption is that the current level of congressional management of both the program in its entirety and FFS Medicare will continue for the foreseeable future. That assumption makes us skeptical that, in the current environment, Congress will allow FFS Medicare to become a prudent purchaser of health-care services. Competitive pricing would change that environment.

2

Five Ways to Pay Medicare Health Plans

Given that the program currently offers—and *should* offer—a public plan and private plans, Medicare faces the question of how to pay those plans efficiently and fairly. We think competitive pricing is the best way to pay all Medicare health plans. To understand why competitive pricing is preferable to the proposed alternatives, it will be helpful first to understand the weaknesses of the alternatives.

MA Payment Policy through 2008

Since 2006, MA plans have bid to offer parts A and B coverage to beneficiaries. (Bids for Part D prescription drug coverage are collected separately.)[1] The plans' bids are based on a beneficiary with average health status and include plan administrative costs and profit.[2] The bids are compared against a benchmark. As described by MedPAC:

> The benchmark is an administratively determined bidding target. [The 1997 BBA] established benchmarks in each county, which included a floor—a minimum amount below which no county benchmarks could go. By design, the floor rate exceeded FFS spending in many counties. It was established to attract plans to areas (mostly rural) with lower-than-average FFS spending. Legislation in 2000 established a second, higher "urban" floor, which applied only to counties in metropolitan areas with more than 250,000 residents. Also, no benchmark can be below per capita FFS spending in a county. (U.S. Medicare Payment Advisory Commission 2008a, 245)

31

Under the provisions of the MMA, annual increases in the benchmark are set at the highest of three adjustments: 2 percent growth, the national growth rate in per-capita Medicare spending, or the growth rate in FFS expenditures for the county. These formulas were imposed on top of previous adjustments that had increased county-level benchmarks relative to FFS expenditures in large, urban counties and other, mostly rural counties to encourage HMO participation in those areas.[3] The result of these methods has been to set MA payment rates at least as high as FFS costs, and often substantially higher.

Plans bidding above the benchmark receive the benchmark payment and are required to charge beneficiaries an additional premium equal to the difference between the benchmark and the plan's bid. Plans bidding below the benchmark are paid their bid plus 75 percent of the difference between the bid and the benchmark—which the plan must return to beneficiaries as supplemental benefits, lower Part B premiums, or lower cost-sharing. On average in 2007, MA enrollees received $86 per month of extra benefits, mainly in the form of buy-downs of Part B cost-sharing (U.S. Department of Health and Human Services, Centers for Medicare and Medicaid Services 2007).

MedPAC assessed the current state of the program as a tradeoff between access and cost (U.S. Medicare Payment Advisory Commission 2008a). As a result of higher payment rates in 2008, all Medicare beneficiaries have access to an MA plan, with an average of thirty-five plans in each county. Eighty-five percent have access to a local HMO or preferred provider organization, and all beneficiaries have a private fee-for-service plan available. But in 2008, the payments to MA plans exceeded those of FFS Medicare (which, we again emphasize, is a questionable standard for efficiency) by 13 percent on average. For 2009, MedPAC estimates payments to exceed FFS Medicare by 14 percent (U.S. Medicare Payment Advisory Commission 2009). "This added cost contributes to the worsening long-range financial sustainability of the Medicare program," according to MedPAC (U.S. Medicare Payment Advisory Commission 2008a, 238). In addition, some quality measures show disappointing levels of quality in MA plans, with slower rates of improvement than for commercial and Medicaid plans. Virtually no quality data at all, however, are available on the most important standard of comparison for MA plans—FFS Medicare.

MedPAC has found that high benchmarks subvert the original conception of having private plans in Medicare, which was to introduce innovation and competition with FFS Medicare (albeit only on the basis of benefits, not premiums) while saving taxpayers a modicum of money. Bids by the most rapidly growing type of MA plan, the private FFS plans, averaged 108 percent of FFS expenditures in 2008. MedPAC notes: "Paying a [private health] plan more than FFS spending is not an efficient use of Medicare funds, particularly if the payments do not result in improved quality of care" (U.S. Medicare Payment Advisory Commission 2008a, 248). Interestingly, MedPAC has not objected to "overpaying" FFS Medicare in areas with high FFS costs relative to private plans, even though FFS has no *demonstrated* quality advantage to justify the difference.

As a result of generous payments, zero-premium MA plans are found in almost all areas of the country and are available to 86 percent of all Medicare beneficiaries (U.S. Department of Health and Human Services, Centers for Medicare and Medicaid Services 2007). But what is the policy justification for this "blanket the country" approach, apart from creating an entitlement to a free MA plan similar to the entitlement to FFS Medicare at no cost beyond the Part B premium? From a cost perspective, this payment system is unsustainable. It is also unfair in that MA plans in areas with high FFS costs offer generous free supplementary benefits to beneficiaries, while beneficiaries in areas with lower FFS costs must pay out of pocket for the same benefits.

Some, largely from the health plan industry (in, for example, America's Health Insurance Plans 2007), claim that higher MA payments are justified because MA plans provide an important option for low-income and minority beneficiaries. Certainly, as documented by Thorpe and Atherly (2002), MA plans in areas of high FFS costs have been able to provide generous and free supplementary benefits valued highly by low-income beneficiaries. This approach to assisting low-income beneficiaries is, however, both inefficient and grossly unfair. First, why should assistance be offered to both wealthy and poor beneficiaries in areas with high FFS costs? It would be more efficient to stop overpaying MA plans and target the assistance only to the needy. Second, why should only those low-income beneficiaries living in areas of high FFS Medicare costs receive such assistance? If low-income beneficiaries need additional assistance beyond that offered through Medicaid, subsidies for Part D plans, and other subsidies, wouldn't it be fairer to offer the same level of subsidy to all qualified low-income beneficiaries nationwide, not solely to those who happen to live in areas with high FFS Medicare costs?

Private fee-for-service (PFFS) plans present a special problem in MA reimbursement. They receive payments through the same methodology as other MA plans, but their payments lack much of the same justification. MedPAC notes:

> PFFS plans do not have provider networks, and they pay providers at Medicare rates—that is, they operate like traditional FFS. However, they are less efficient than the traditional FFS program; they bid 8 percent higher than FFS for the same benefit package. PFFS plans have fewer program requirements than coordinated care plans; the law exempts them from the quality reporting requirements applicable to other plan types. An additional concern is that PFFS plans and their brokers have been responsible for a large portion of the marketing abuses in the MA program, which have resulted in sanctions and fines from the Centers for Medicare & Medicaid Services (CMS), including a moratorium on marketing and sanctions and fines on brokers by the states. (U.S. Medicare Payment Advisory Commission 2008a, 243)

Of the MA growth in 2007, 60 percent occurred in PFFS plans (U.S. Medicare Payment Advisory Commission 2008a). As a result, a large part of the increase in payments to MA plans is being made to the plans with the least policy justification.[4]

MedPAC's Proposal: Set MA Payments Equal to Average County-Level FFS Spending

MedPAC has argued long and forcefully that paying private plans more than FFS Medicare makes little economic or policy sense:

> The Commission supports private plans in the Medicare program. Beneficiaries should be able to choose between the FFS

Medicare program and the alternative delivery systems that private plans can provide.[5] Private plans may use care management techniques, and—if paid appropriately—they have the incentive to innovate.

However, the Commission also supports financial neutrality between payment rates for the FFS program and the MA program. Financial neutrality means that the Medicare program *should pay the same amount regardless of which Medicare option a beneficiary chooses.* Neutrality is important to restore the original goal of having private plans in Medicare: to stimulate efficiency and innovation. Currently, the MA system increases government outlays and beneficiary premiums (including those who elect to remain in traditional Medicare) at a time when Medicare is under increasing financial stress. (U.S. Medicare Payment Advisory Commission 2008a, 248; emphasis added)

MedPAC projected government payments to private plans for 2009 to be 114 percent of corresponding FFS levels, a slight increase from 2008 (U.S. Medicare Payment Advisory Commission 2009). On average, HMOs were estimated to provide traditional Part A and Part B services for 99 percent of FFS expenditures, while the corresponding PFFS plan bids averaged 108 percent of FFS expenditures. MedPAC reached a clear conclusion:

We are concerned that the average MA bid for Medicare Part A and Part B services is above average FFS spending. This means that, on average,[6] all extra services by the plan are funded by the Medicare program and not by plan efficiencies. In addition, a significant portion of the value of the extra benefits goes to fund plan administration and profits and not to services for beneficiaries.

The MA program as currently structured does not ensure that any added benefits are delivered as efficiently as possible. Many MA plans have demonstrably higher costs than traditional Medicare. Moreover, increasing MA payments in low-cost areas does little to reward the providers responsible for keeping down costs in those areas. A better approach would be to reward

providers in low-cost areas through the FFS payment structure—
or better yet, through innovative new payment systems.

By increasing payment to levels significantly above traditional Medicare, we have changed the signal we are sending to
the market: Instead of efficiency-enhancing innovation, we are
getting plans (private FFS) that are much like traditional Medicare, except at a higher cost. (U.S. Medicare Payment Advisory
Commission 2008a, 248)

By changing the government payment to FFS levels, Medicare no longer
would subsidize private plans that can't match FFS costs, much less
improve on FFS delivery methods. But it is worth noting that while Med-
PAC's proposal certainly would save money, it does not go far enough.
According to MedPAC, Medicare "should pay the same amount regardless
of which Medicare option a beneficiary chooses." In that event, it matters
entirely what the "same amount" will be. If the amount is set using FFS
costs, the new payment system will create a new set of winners and losers,
depending on how generous FFS payment levels are in relation to the unre-
vealed costs of private plans.

This is the adjusted average per-capita cost (AAPCC) method all over
again,[7] albeit

- with better risk-adjustment methods today than when the
  AAPCC originally was employed;

- without the 5 percent discount applied to HMO payments; and

- without some of the benefit inefficiencies of the old AAPCC
  system.[8]

Dowd, Coulam, and Feldman note that it was "difficult to find any ana-
lyst who [expressed] a positive view of [the AAPCC] system" (2000, 9). Yet,
under MedPAC's current proposal, we would return to that flawed system.
It is worth reflecting on why that is a bad idea.

The basic concept behind the AAPCC was to link the payment of
HMOs in each county to a discounted estimate of the costs of FFS beneficiaries in that county, standardized for the risk status of the beneficiaries.

The AAPCC payment was generally equal to 95 percent of the standardized FFS costs per FFS beneficiary in the county (computed separately for aged and disabled beneficiaries, and separately for Medicare parts A and B). Payments for specific enrollees involved simple multiplication of the AAPCC base rate for each county by the risk adjustment that applied to each enrollee. HMOs contracting with Medicare were required to submit reports to establish each HMO's so-called adjusted community rate (ACR) for each county. The ACR was the amount it would cost the plan to provide basic entitlement services to Medicare enrollees while earning the same rate of return as for commercial enrollees. If the ACR showed HMO costs below the AAPCC, the HMO was required to return the difference to the government or (as did most plans) to beneficiaries in the form of added benefits or reduced cost-sharing.

Risk adjustment was based on crude demographic attributes, including gender, age, institutional status, work status, and Medicaid status, and it entered the payment calculation in both factors: computation of the standardized base rate for each county, and the adjustment to that base rate for each enrollee, based on demographic traits. There were very serious problems with this system.

Substantial Variation in Payments. AAPCC amounts varied substantially by area. The differences among geographically proximate counties were a curiosity, but the regional differences were staggering. In the mid-1990s, for example, Medicare reimbursement per enrollee was $8,537 in Miami but only $3,300 in Minneapolis (Skinner and Fisher 1997). This dramatic variation raised questions about the legitimacy of variations in FFS Medicare spending and resulted in vast differences in government-financed benefits for enrollees in private plans, as discussed below.

Variation unrelated to HMO costs. The variation in HMO payments across areas, based on average county-level FFS spending, appeared to be unrelated to the HMOs' costs of providing the entitlement benefit package, as evidenced by the fact that "free" supplementary benefits offered by HMOs varied proportionately with their payment levels (McBride 1998). The variation in average FFS spending also was found to be substantially greater than that in commercial private health plan premiums serving the same areas. Schmid compared AAPCC amounts to HMO premiums in the Federal Employees Health Benefits Program (FEHBP). His key finding was that

> variation of average HMO premiums [in FEHBP] is markedly less than variation of per capita fee-for-service costs as measured by Medicare's adjusted average per capita cost (AAPCC) index. Moreover, average HMO premiums across the [FEHBP] sample were largely uncorrelated with AAPCC values. . . . These findings raise some doubt about the suitability of using the AAPCC index for geographic adjustment of Medicare's HMO capitation payments. (Schmid 1995, 271)

Variation not explained by other factors. As noted by Skinner and Fisher (1997, 414), "There are a number of perfectly good reasons why [payment] disparities exist, including differences in general costs of living, the age structure of the population, and health status. . . . [However, our results show] that even after adjusting for age, sex, race, price, and illness related factors, major variations in Medicare spending persist." And they have persisted since the introduction of the AAPCC (Jencks et al. 2000; Blumberg and Evans 1998).

Generously funded areas getting free extra benefits. Not surprisingly, given variations in the generosity of payments in relation to costs, benefits available to HMO enrollees varied substantially across the country. A system based on FFS costs creates winners and losers without any policy justification for the differences. These de facto outcomes were caused by paying HMOs based on an administrative calculation of the cost of something else (average county-level FFS spending). Medicare beneficiaries in different counties received Medicare benefits of markedly different value. Dowd and others, referring to HMO plans in 2000, noted,

> Medicare beneficiaries in some market areas obtain substantial *government-financed* benefits from [Medicare+Choice] plans— including outpatient prescription drug coverage—at no additional premium. Meanwhile, beneficiaries in other areas pay

substantial premiums for coverage that differs little from the basic entitlement and pay more than $200 per month for M+C drug coverage when it is available at all. (Dowd et al. 2000, 9)

McBride showed in some detail what this meant:

Of particular interest is the large disparity in the availability of plan benefits across different types of counties. For example, whereas 92 percent of beneficiaries are offered prescription drug coverage if they live in a county with an AAPCC rate of $500 or more, this same coverage is available to only 1.9 percent of those living in counties with AAPCC rates below $300. This largely reflects the lower availability of any plan in counties with low AAPCC rates. . . . This suggests that plans that receive higher AAPCC rates are much more likely to be able to afford to cover prescription drugs, often a costly item for aged Medicare enrollees. (McBride 1998, 175)

Inadequate Demographic Risk Adjustment. A number of studies in the 1990s properly pointed out that part of the problem with the AAPCC payment system was inadequate risk adjustment. One justifiable reason for costs to vary from area to area and person to person is that beneficiaries have differing severities of health-care needs, with different cost consequences. According to Newhouse and colleagues, however, the adjusters in the AAPCC formula explained only 1 percent of the variance in actual spending: "On the face of it, 1 percent does not seem like much of an improvement over no risk adjustment at all," they observed, "and, although it is better than nothing, in fact it is not much better." Further, they noted,

The lack of adequate risk adjustment means that the government overpays Medicare managed care plans. . . . Plans have an incentive to attract persons within each class whose expected spending is less than the reimbursement and to dump others. An incentive, of course, may be acted upon to a greater or lesser degree. Although the claim is controversial, our reading of the

> evidence is that plans as a group, not necessarily every plan, have in fact disproportionately attracted beneficiaries whose expected spending is less than 95 percent of AAPCC; thus, there has been favorable selection into plans. (Newhouse et al. 1997, 29)

After the 1990s, following requirements of the Balanced Budget Act, the CMS developed new health-based risk adjustment methods to pay Medicare HMOs. From 2000 through 2003, the agency introduced the principal inpatient diagnostic cost group (PIP-DCG) method, based on Medicare inpatient diagnoses; and beginning in 2004, it implemented the hierarchical condition categories (HCC) method, based on selected significant diagnoses (approximately seventy disease groups for aged/disabled models).

Under industry pressure, data collection requirements were reduced (Weissman et al. 2005). The implementation schedule allowed a gradual transition before HCC methods were fully applied in 2007, but with "budget neutrality" requirements that do not phase out until 2011 (ibid.; U.S. Department of Health and Human Services, Centers for Medicare and Medicaid Services 2007; Pope et al. 2004). Limiting the diagnoses and the scope of data collection reduced the effectiveness of the new method, although it remained a substantial improvement over the one it replaced. As Pope and colleagues wrote:

> In limiting the number of conditions that affect payment, many serious, high-cost diagnoses—especially rare ones—will be ignored. [Managed-care organizations] enrolling beneficiaries with excluded diagnoses will be disadvantaged, and beneficiaries with such conditions may not be well served by MCOs. (Pope et al. 2004, 129)

But perhaps the real question to emphasize when we think about risk adjustment is not how much of the variation in risk is explained by the risk adjuster, but how much more the insurer and the insured know than can ever be explained by the risk adjuster.

Even with the best practical risk adjustment, key problems would remain. First, the cost data on which the AAPCC or its later, more generous equivalents[9] were based are drawn from the costs (higher or lower) of FFS production of the benefit.[10] It is accordingly inevitable that the AAPCC will not track HMO costs in a reliable way. As Blumberg and Evans noted ten years ago:

> There is currently no connection between an individual risk contractor's costs and the capitation rates it receives through the Medicare program, another consequence of linking fee-for-service and HMO payments. This means that in some areas where the AAPCC exceeds HMO costs, the Medicare program has no ability to negotiate lower rates. Conversely, areas where no HMOs participate in the federal program may have AAPCC levels that fall below the plans' costs; in this situation Medicare cannot increase capitation amounts or rates to encourage participation— even if these higher costs were determined to be at an efficient level. (Blumberg and Evans 1998, 65)

Any AAPCC-like system will continue to have areas where FFS and MA plans are "overpaid" and "underpaid" without any policy justification. This result is an artifact of the *intrinsic limits* of any such method that estimates HMO payments from FFS costs.

These arbitrary variations are especially important given that the system uses the county as the unit of geographic adjustment. Even if a collection of counties sums to a reasonable notion of the "market area," the inconsistency of AAPCC-style payments means "border issues" will inevitably arise. "Because HMO service areas can span more than one county," Blumberg and Evans wrote, "an HMO has an incentive to avoid Medicare beneficiaries living in counties with low payment rates and to recruit heavily from counties with high payment rates" (1998, 67). The geographic units for the payment calculation could be changed, but as long as the base payment rates for geographic units are computed directly from FFS costs for beneficiaries in those units, the difficulty will remain.

Continued Inefficiency Despite "Cost Savings." While saving money compared with the current payment system,[11] MedPAC's proposal would continue to pay more than the costs of the most efficient qualified health plan in high MA payment areas. It is unclear to us why the government should pay any health plan more than it costs efficient health plans to deliver the entitlement benefits. When payment arrangements create a patchwork of overpayments that have no intrinsic justification, some beneficiaries will receive free benefits. But this comes at the expense of taxpayers, who can ill afford such generosity; and, to use MedPAC's phrase, it "contributes to the worsening long-range financial sustainability of the Medicare program" (U.S. Medicare Payment Advisory Commission 2008a, 238).

Berenson notes that "the benchmarks against which MA plans bid do not reflect appropriate targets because they do not reflect cost differences faced by local plans as a result of local market factors but rather are artifacts of the specific cost factors faced by the traditional Medicare program" (2008, w160). MedPAC appears to acknowledge that FFS costs are not necessarily an appropriate benchmark:

> We want to be clear that even though we use the FFS Medicare spending level as a measure of parity for the MA program, this should not be taken as a conclusion that the Commission believes that FFS Medicare is an efficient delivery system in most markets. In fact, much of our work is devoted to identifying inefficiencies in FFS Medicare and suggesting improvements in the program. However, good policy might argue that coordinated care systems found in many MA plans should always be able to be as efficient as FFS Medicare and in most cases should be more efficient. We would also like to note that some level of inefficiency is built into benchmarks based on FFS spending. (U.S. Medicare Payment Advisory Commission 2008a, 248)

Our argument is in this spirit. But we take an evenhanded view of the inefficiency that results from overpayment. We oppose overpayment of either MA plans or FFS Medicare. We are concerned that MedPAC's proposal is not sustainable in the long run, and that it will create overpaid "winning" counties that will look just as unjustifiable in a few years (after this latter-day AAPCC is introduced) as they did in 1997—indeed worse, because the fiscal constraints of Medicare are likely to be far more pronounced. Moreover, this approach is bad economic policy for exactly the reason MedPAC cites in its critique of the current payment system: It signals to the market that payment is not tied directly to efficiency and low costs.

A second approach would be to adjust MA payments by using some additional source of data from which to infer what Medicare should pay. This approach is the essence of the proposal by Robert Berenson, described next.

Berenson's Proposal: Adjust MA Payments
Using MA Cost Reports and Other Data

Robert Berenson, MD, is one of the nation's most knowledgeable experts on Medicare payments and health plans.[12] Berenson accepts the weakness of the MedPAC option and frames a solution of analytical adjustments to FFS costs that comes just short of competitive bidding for private plans.

For Berenson, while MA payment reform will reduce payments in any event, it matters how the specific payment approach produces different relative losers. He frames the problem as how to set county-level benchmarks responsive to local market factors that affect private plans' costs:

> Whether private plans, functioning under current market conditions that often favor providers' pricing power, or traditional Medicare, hampered by congressional micromanagement, is more successful at restraining inflationary cost pressures—or, more precisely, less unsuccessful—is an empirical question. . . .
> I take the position that paying the MA and traditional Medicare sectors equitably actually requires adjusting traditional Medicare payment levels to recognize how local market costs for health plans vary. (Berenson 2008, w157, 158)

The great virtue of Berenson's discussion is to show the limitations of tying the benchmarks to FFS costs and to suggest an analytical strategy for adjusting those benchmarks to reflect local market factors. The strategy is based on the "bids" MA plans now submit. Currently, these bids have no effect on the establishment of the benchmark—when MA plans bid, they know what the benchmark is (currently well above the FFS cost in most counties). Berenson proposes to use the actuarial estimates supporting the bids as a platform for statistical analyses to estimate how local MA costs vary in relation to FFS costs:

> For purposes of the needed analysis that focuses on relative bids across geographic areas, plan bids generally reflect the costs of efficiently providing Medicare benefits. . . . By reviewing all bids from each county for all MA plans except PFFS plans, one can determine how costs in plans vary geographically and how well, using formal statistical techniques, that variation correlates with the variation in spending at the county level in traditional Medicare. (Ibid., w161)

To the degree that local MA costs vary more or less than FFS costs, the benchmark would be adjusted accordingly—down for counties in which MA bids reveal costs below FFS, up in largely rural or small urban areas without much competition where MA bids are above FFS levels. This would be done through the device of blending national and local per-capita spending levels.

Taken to the extreme, Berenson's approach would be roughly equivalent to treating actuarial data submitted by MA plans (the "adjusted community rates," or ACRs) as bids, in an MA plan–only competitive pricing system (an approach that, conceptually, at least, is not very different from President Obama's proposal, described as the fifth option below). But Berenson does not, explicitly at least, push the adjustments that far. He appears to view his approach more modestly, as a way to address the MedPAC proposal's main weakness: its failure to tie payments to MA plan costs. He emphasizes both the need for more analysis to determine the consistency of the relationship between plan costs and FFS spending and the need to bear in mind how this proposal would moderate MedPAC's payment reductions in many areas. Indeed, the net effect of his proposal would be that "rural and lower-cost urban areas—many in the Northern Tier—would do better than under MedPAC's preferred formulation" (Ibid., w162).

Many variants on Berenson's proposals could be imagined—for instance, introducing other data into the adjustments. But his proposals stand for the most refined form of setting MA payment rates using administrative data in that they don't construe a "level playing field" in nearly so simple a way as does MedPAC, and they urge a conversation on what, politically, we actually want to level—even though Berenson recognizes that any approach (his or MedPAC's) that reforms MA payments will create losers and set off, in the process, a "geographically based Congressional 'food fight'" (Ibid., w162).

The critical question, we think, is whether going down the road of "adjustments" is a sound strategy. On this, two points should be noted. First, like the MA-only bidding models he rightly criticizes, Berenson's proposal would leave traditional Medicare "undisciplined." To be sure, in areas where MA costs are above FFS levels, the adjustments proposed by MedPAC would be moderated; in that sense, FFS would be less attractive in those areas, and private plans would be more likely to serve them. But in other areas where MA plans are more efficient than FFS, his methods would reduce MA payments below FFS levels while leaving FFS reimbursement untouched.

Second, it is worth emphasizing again the key problem of having the government establish "adjustments." It is the generic problem of using administrative methods to set prices. As emphasized by Dowd and others in a discussion of what were then termed Medicare+Choice (M+C) plans:

> The most glaring problem with the current payment system [AAPCC] . . . is that information about the costs of care flows in the wrong direction: from the organization that knows very little about M+C costs (the federal government) to the organizations that know as much as possible (the M+C plans). A common response to the problems of the current administrative payment system is some form of competitive pricing.
>
> Competitive pricing reverses the flow of cost information; that is, M+C plans tell the government how much it costs to care for Medicare beneficiaries. Plans submit bids under a system that rewards low bids and penalizes high bids. An important distinction between competitive pricing and the current payment system is that rewards and penalties are linked primarily to the prices submitted by plans, rather than to the level of benefits they provide. (Dowd et al. 2000, 10)

This homily from Economics 100 remains the most compelling justification for a competitive pricing approach that avoids "adjustment" strategies. We turn now to that approach.

Competitive Pricing

All of the pricing methods outlined above rely on manipulations of administrative data by the Centers for Medicare and Medicaid Services. Unfortunately, these administrative pricing methods do not reliably reveal the costs of efficient plans in each area.

There simply is no economic justification for Congress to act as the administrative rate-setter. A more logical approach to determine the price of the entitlement benefit package is *to ask the health plans how much it costs*. Their incentive to tell the truth is higher out-of-pocket premiums for higher-priced plans, and premium rebates or enhanced benefits for lower-priced plans. Under competitive pricing, the government would substitute market-like arrangements for the administrative calculations the CMS has traditionally used to set payments to private plans.[13] The design comprises four major elements (described in more detail in Dowd and Feldman 2002):

- *Eligibility and participation of plans.* The CMS would, as it does now, require that private plans report quality measures and meet minimum levels of quality before allowing them to participate in Medicare.[14]

- *Benefit package.* Congress would determine a national entitlement benefit package (for example, the current benefits or an expanded entitlement package).

- *Structure and conduct of the bidding process.* Private health plans and FFS Medicare would submit bids on the entitlement benefits for a standardized enrollee in each market area. (Private plans would choose their service areas; FFS Medicare would serve all areas.)

- *Determination of government payments from the bids.* The government premium contribution for all plans including FFS

Medicare would be set as a function of the risk-adjusted bids of the qualified health plans able to enroll some minimum proportion of the beneficiaries in the local area. (Plans able to serve only marginal numbers of enrollees would not set the benchmark for all plans.) We prefer for the government to set its premium contribution at the lowest risk-adjusted bid of a qualified plan, subject to capacity limits.

Under competitive pricing, beneficiaries would have guaranteed access to all health plans in their market areas at annual open-enrollment periods. The FFS "bid" would be the federal government's best estimate of the cost of providing the entitlement benefit package to a standardized beneficiary in each county in the United States. FFS Medicare would be available in all market areas, but it would have to charge an additional premium if its bid exceeded the premium of the lowest priced plan in an area. If deemed appropriate, the special obligations of FFS Medicare, including universal availability and subsidies for medical education or facilities that treat a disproportionate share of low-income patients, could be acknowledged by adjustments to the FFS bid.[15] If no MA plans were available in a market area, then FFS Medicare would be the default plan, and it would be available for the Part B premium.

Under our proposal, beneficiaries living in different parts of the country would pay different amounts for FFS Medicare, and for private plans. Although this may seem objectionable, there is a strong precedent for making some beneficiaries pay more than others for FFS Medicare. By introducing means-tested Part B premiums for high-income beneficiaries in 2007, Congress already has determined that this can happen without violating the original intent of the program. The current differentiation is based on the beneficiary's income. Our proposal introduces a second differentiation—whether a private health plan is available in the market area that can offer the basic benefit package at lower cost than FFS Medicare.

Competitive pricing addresses inefficiency caused by distorted prices in the Medicare program. When Congress (representing both taxpayers and currently eligible beneficiaries) bases its decisions about entitlement benefits on the administered prices of those benefits, rather than prices in the most efficient health plan in each market area, those prices will be too high in some market areas. As a result, Congress will set the benefit package too low, excluding some benefits for which taxpayers and beneficiaries would pay willingly at the efficient prices.

Evidence of FFS Medicare's unwillingness to add new benefits can be seen in a number of areas, including outpatient prescription drug benefits, which were a standard feature of private health insurance plans before Medicare offered Part D in 2006. Medicare also lagged behind the private sector in covering preventive services. For example, pap smears and glaucoma screening were not covered until 2000—years after the private sector started covering these important screening tools. Medicare's tardiness may be explained by the cost of adding this coverage. If benefits that taxpayers and beneficiaries want at the efficient prices could be offered for those prices, Congress might be more inclined to add them. We believe that competitive pricing can determine the efficient prices, and, in many areas, these will be less than the cost in FFS Medicare.

Competitive pricing could have a substantial effect on the amounts the government pays to health plans in many areas. We estimate the overall savings from a competitive pricing system in chapter 4 below. To get some idea of the potential effects of competitive pricing, note the results of the aborted 1997 demonstration of competitive pricing for private Medicare plans only in Denver to replace AAPCC payments. The bids submitted by four private plans for the entitlement benefit package were 25–38 percent lower than the government's payments to the plans at that time (Dowd 2001). Why should competitive bidding produce such savings? The answer appears simple. In Denver, the basic benefit package cost less to produce than the AAPCC, but the AAPCC did not have any procedural way to obtain that information or adjust prices for it. The threat to high bidders of having to charge substantial out-of-pocket premiums for basic benefits and the opportunity for low bidders to provide additional benefits or lower premiums created strong incentives for Denver plans to submit low bids.[16]

Any discussion of bidding raises the question, "On what should health plans bid?" Our answer is, "The entitlement benefit package." But, as noted earlier, we would alter the definition of the entitlement benefit package to include only those features required of all participating plans, because those are the ones that should be viewed as necessary to accomplish the purposes of the Medicare program for all beneficiaries. Critics of competitive pricing are likely to focus on two features of FFS Medicare that are not required of MA plans, features that would be converted from statutory entitlements to supplementary benefits in competitive pricing as we have defined it: open access to providers and a national service area.

Open Access. "Open access" means that beneficiaries can see, without a referral and without any substantial utilization controls, any health-care provider who accepts Medicare terms. Is that plan feature properly considered part of the entitlement, or is it a supplementary benefit? We offer a two-part response to the question.

First, MA plans typically do not feature the same level of open access as FFS Medicare. They have provider networks and employ at least modest restrictions on access and utilization, such as differential copayments for in-network and out-of-network providers. The same is true of most commercial insurance plans and some public programs (such as Medicaid). The most popular health plan in the commercial health insurance market is the preferred provider organization (PPO), in which consumers have financial incentives to use certain doctors who are selected by the plan. Open access as in Medicare FFS, where beneficiaries can see any participating provider without a referral, is a supplementary benefit that is worth less than its cost to covered employees and dependents. By requiring open access only of FFS Medicare and then setting the benchmark at least as high as FFS costs, Congress is paying for a form of coverage that is a supplementary benefit in today's commercial health insurance market.

Second, critics might argue that open access, attainable for no more than the Part B premium, needs to be preserved for low-income beneficiaries. But as noted earlier, Thorpe and Atherly (2002) have shown that low-income beneficiaries disproportionately decline the open-access features of FFS Medicare when offered better benefits in MA plans. If maintaining the status quo (better benefits *and* low premiums) for low-income beneficiaries is a priority, then means-tested subsidies (that is, portable vouchers) for the poor that are the same regardless of the health plan chosen are a far more efficient approach than overpaying FFS Medicare for all beneficiaries in the market area.

In our competitive pricing proposal, Congress could continue to require that FFS Medicare offer open access, perhaps because Congress believes that at least one health plan in Medicare should have that feature. That is a perfectly legitimate rationale for imposing that feature on FFS Medicare; but if open access makes FFS Medicare more expensive than private plans, beneficiaries should pay for that supplementary benefit out of their own pockets. Alternatively, Congress could allow FFS Medicare to offer plan options that utilize selective provider contracting and more limited access to specialists.

National Service Area. By "national service area," we mean that care from all providers is covered to the same extent, regardless of their locations relative to the beneficiary's place of residence. All MA plans are required to make arrangements for short-term coverage of emergency care outside their much smaller local or regional service areas and provider networks, but only FFS Medicare offers long-term coverage of nonemergency services in all areas nationwide.[17] The universal coverage requirement means that FFS Medicare must pay a claim for covered services obtained from any participating provider anywhere in the United States. Some additional cost is likely to be associated with that requirement.

Again, we offer a two-part response. First, we emphasize that a national service area for nonemergency services is limited in the commercial insurance market and Medicaid programs. Commercial insurance plans usually allow out-of-network coverage for a fee; Medicaid is more restrictive, permitting out-of-state coverage only for emergency services. Second, low-income Medicare beneficiaries tend to reject the national service area in FFS Medicare in favor of other benefits offered by MA plans.

In our competitive pricing proposal, Congress could continue to require FFS Medicare to offer a national service area, but if that supplementary benefit resulted in FFS Medicare being more expensive than private plans, beneficiaries would have to pay for it out of their own pockets. Alternatively, Congress could allow FFS Medicare to offer plan options for covering out-of-area services that mirror the out-of-network coverage of MA plans. MA beneficiaries who reside in different locations for substantial amounts of time during the year could enroll in a private fee-for-service (PFFS) plan or an MA plan that has an "extended absence option."

The Obama Proposal: MA-Only Bidding

During his campaign and transition, President Obama made no secret of his intention to cut payments to MA plans. For example, as he noted shortly after his election, "The Medicare Advantage program is one that I've already cited where we're spending billions of dollars subsidizing insurance companies for a program that doesn't appreciably improve the health of seniors under Medicare. So our starting point is savings" (Reichard 2008). Once in office, his administration moved quickly to reduce MA payments for 2010 through changes in payment formulae (for example, see U.S. Department of Health and Human Services, Centers for Medicare and Medicaid Services 2009 and Fuhrmans and Zhang 2009). The administration also announced a plan for competitive bidding:

> For years we've been paying Medicare Advantage plans 14 percent more than it would cost for the traditional Medicare plan. In this budget, we have a simple idea: Instead of government setting prices for our seniors, why not have private plans bid for Medicare's business? This competitive bidding is good for businesses, it's good for our seniors, and it's good for taxpayers, because it saves us $177 billion over 10 years. (Obama 2009)

The administration's competitive bidding plans were proposed as part of a ten-year budget blueprint. Details of the competitive pricing program are sketchy at this writing, but the essential structure appears to be as follows:

- "The final proposal is expected to call for a two-year 'phasedown'— in 2011 and 2012—of rates paid to MA carriers to reach 100% of traditional Medicare fee-for-service (FFS)" (Davis, 2009).

- In 2013, MA plans will participate in a competitive-bidding process. FFS will be excluded from the bidding.

- The geographic unit of bidding is not yet clear—whether counties, as at present, or some larger aggregation.[18]

- Plans will submit bids based on a standardized benefit package.

- The benchmark price will be based on the weighted average of the bids submitted, with the weights based on enrollment the previous year (Carr 2009). When details are worked out, the proposal may include a restriction on bids—for example, requiring that benchmarks be no more than current benchmarks or FFS spending levels.[19]

- It is expected that plans whose bids exceed the benchmark will be required to charge a premium. It is unclear whether plans bidding below the benchmark will receive all of the difference (currently, MA plans bidding below the benchmark receive 75 percent of the difference), and under what terms (for example, a requirement to convert the difference to premium reductions, benefit enhancements, or quality improvements).

As noted earlier, this constitutes a major change from current bidding practices in which the bids have no effect on the benchmark. We agree entirely with President Obama's "simple idea" of having plans submit bids to set prices. The devil here is in one large matter and certain details.

The big flaw is the exclusion of FFS from the bidding system. This may be a form of political expedience, although we don't know that. But an "MA-only" design has serious problems. The Obama model is little different from the MA-only competitive bidding design that the CMS attempted to demonstrate in the 1990s. As Berenson has noted of that experience:

> In the context of [1990s competitive pricing demonstrations], the Association of Health Insurance Plans (AHIP) argued, with justification, that the competitive pricing design was tilted in favor of traditional (FFS) Medicare because plans bidding only against each other would face pricing discipline from market competition, whereas the traditional program would effectively be given a pass. Under that bidding approach, only beneficiaries selecting the traditional Medicare program would continue to be highly subsidized for their selection. (2008, w161)

Berenson went on to say that

without a consensus on what constitutes a level playing field—
indeed, even whether there should be a level playing field—this
former CMS model of competitive pricing would appear off the
table currently. (Ibid.)

An MA-only bidding model thus is likely to provoke serious political
problems of its own, given the "unbalanced playing field" it creates. But
President Obama has put it back on the table and is attempting to build a
consensus for it.

Quite apart from the politics of the proposal, its economics are trou-
bling. The inefficiency that results from excluding FFS is not small. In areas
where FFS is more expensive than the MA plans, beneficiaries who prefer
FFS will not have to weigh that preference against the fact that FFS costs
the Medicare program more money. There will be no price signal to encourage them to choose the cheaper option, even when the additional cost of
FFS isn't worth the extra money *to beneficiaries*—an excellent criterion for
determining when Medicare shouldn't pay the extra money. The reverse
also is true, depending on the bidding rules:[20] In areas where FFS is
cheaper, beneficiaries who prefer MA plans will not have to pay the extra
cost their preference imposes on the program, a cost that may not be worth
it to beneficiaries. At a time when Medicare faces extreme financial pressure, *this is bad policy*.

Apart from these inefficiencies, the president's proposal makes an
additional, unfortunate choice in using the average of all bids to set the
benchmark. Chapter 4 below provides estimates of the savings to be
obtained from competitive pricing. One message of that chapter is that
using the average of all bids, rather than the lowest qualified bid, is likely
to reduce substantially the savings from competitive pricing. The president's choice of a benchmark may make the bidding system more politically palatable, but it costs money at a time when the program is in a
financial crisis.

For these reasons, the Obama plan appears to create serious political
and economic problems without many compensating benefits. We believe
the economic case for including FFS is overwhelming. As to the possible
political difficulties of including FFS and setting the benchmark at the low
bidder, we urge readers to suspend judgment until:

- Chapter 4—The data we will present here suggest that certain common understandings of competitive pricing may be erroneous—specifically, the assumption that it will impose additional costs on the order of, say, 10 percent or more on current FFS enrollees if FFS is included in the bidding. In fact, we will show that relatively few beneficiaries will face disruptions that large.

- Chapters 6 and 8—These chapters will suggest that policies to buffer a transition (such as hold-harmless provisions that phase down over a fixed period of time) can be implemented so that beneficiaries are not unduly disrupted in areas where FFS enrollment will result in large cost increases.

We are well aware of the generally dismal political history of competitive pricing in Medicare (chapter 6). But, given the seriousness of the current financial crisis, the benefits of competitive pricing for public and private plans, and the possibility of practical remedies to ease beneficiaries through a transition, the Obama proposals are an unsatisfying half a loaf.

3

Technical Issues in Competitive
Pricing for Medicare

In this chapter, we discuss several technical issues to clarify what we mean by bringing competitive pricing to Medicare. We begin by explaining the current payment arrangements for three types of MA plans—local coordinated care plans, regional preferred provider organizations, and private fee-for-service plans. Since these arrangements involve a form of bidding, albeit against known benchmarks that do not depend on plans' bids, we ask whether plans' bids in the current bidding system reflect their costs. The answer to this question will affect our estimate of the savings from competitive pricing in the following chapter.

The short answer to our question is a qualified, "Yes," but the qualifications are important. Exclusion of FFS Medicare from the current system—which implies that MA plans can give premium rebates, but they cannot force FFS to charge more than the Part B premium—may weaken the MA plans' motivation to submit low bids. We also contrast bidding against a known benchmark in the current system with our proposal for determining the benchmark from the plans' bids themselves—a fundamental distinction.

In the second part of the chapter, we compare different ways of setting the government premium contribution. We suggest that, despite some theory-based predictions to the contrary, setting the contribution equal to the second-lowest bid would not save money for Medicare compared with our proposal for setting the contribution equal to the lowest bid. We recommend that the government contribution be set equal to the lowest bid from a qualified plan. We review some concerns that typically arise when the contribution is based on the lowest bid and argue that those concerns are unjustified. Indeed, we think these concerns, as expressed, are in most cases likely to be red herrings, and we recommend that the government be wary of rejecting any bids that seem "unreasonably" low.

Current Payment Arrangements

There are two types of private health plans in Medicare, distinguished by the size of their services areas. "Local" coordinated care plans (mainly HMOs) are private plans that can enter Medicare on a county-by-county basis and receive a predetermined payment from the program for each enrollee. Regional preferred provider organizations (PPOs) agree to cover one or more of twenty-six geographic regions defined by the CMS (instead of defining their own service areas, county by county, as local plans do). Payment for regional PPOs is determined in the same way as that for local plans, except the benchmarks are calculated differently (U.S. Medicare Payment Advisory Commission 2008b). The regional benchmark is a weighted average of the average county rate for the region and the average plan bid. Consequently (and unlike in the payment system for local plans), the benchmark for regional PPOs is based in part on plan bids. This would be a more important and promising method if the regional PPOs had more substantial enrollments—according to the Kaiser Family Foundation (2008), only 3 percent of Medicare Advantage enrollees were enrolled in regional PPOs in 2008—and if the weight given to plan bids, as opposed to the predetermined rates, were greater.[1]

Private fee-for-service (PFFS) plans submit a single bid but can define their own service areas. Because they disproportionately choose to operate in counties where benchmarks are high relative to FFS costs, PFFS plans have one of the highest ratios of plan payments to FFS expenditures, estimated by MedPAC at 120 percent in 2008 (U.S. Senate, Committee on Finance 2008).

Do MA Plans' Current "Bids" Reflect Their Costs?

If MA plans' bids in the current system are close to their costs, then the competitive pricing system we propose will not have much effect on those bids. Under the current payment system, plans that submit high bids might have to charge out-of-pocket premiums, depending on the county-level benchmarks, while those that submit low bids compared with the benchmark can offer premium rebates or provide extra benefits. The opportunity to give rebates or extra benefits and the penalty for high bids should provide an incentive for plans to submit bids that are close to their costs. These features of the payment system would not change under our proposal. But rather than bidding against a known benchmark, plans in our proposal would be bidding against an unknown benchmark based on the plans' bids, and bids below the benchmark would not be subject to a 25 percent tax. Moreover, private health plans would be in direct price competition with FFS Medicare and have an opportunity for a substantial increase in their market shares.

To project plans' bids in a competitive pricing system, the U.S. Congressional Budget Office (2006) assumed that plans' bids equaled their costs, as reported in the ACR submissions of plans that participated in Medicare in 2005. The CBO justified using ACR data as follows: "The Medicare Advantage payment system gives plans an incentive to provide Medicare benefits efficiently because the lower a plan's cost of providing those benefits relative to the benchmark, the greater the additional benefits or premium rebates it can offer to beneficiaries" (ibid., 36–37).[2] Several features of the current bidding system may affect plans' motivations to submit low bids, however.

Exclusion of FFS. The first feature is the exclusion of FFS Medicare from the current bidding system. A private plan that submits a low bid can offer rebates or additional benefits that attract enrollees from FFS, but no matter what it bids, it cannot make FFS enrollees pay more than the Part B premium. The exclusion of FFS from competitive bidding was a focal point of health plans' objections to the Denver demonstration (Dowd, Coulam, and Feldman 2000). The question of how to include FFS in a competitive pricing system has long been debated. It is worth reviewing that history to explain why plans' bids might actually be different in the system we propose.

The Balanced Budget Act of 1997 (BBA, Public Law 105-33), which authorized the HCFA (later the CMS) to demonstrate competitive payment systems for Medicare+Choice organizations, made no reference to demonstrating competitive pricing for traditional FFS Medicare. Based on the recommendation of its Competitive Pricing Advisory Committee (CPAC), the HCFA's design for the demonstration excluded FFS Medicare. CPAC had reservations about excluding FFS. As expressed in its *Design Report*:

> The CPAC was advised that the intent of the demonstration was to develop a pricing methodology for Medicare+Choice organizations only. But the committee urged HCFA to explore the receptivity of Congress to include fee-for-service in the demonstration. The committee also expressed the judgment that the exclusion of fee-for-service might jeopardize the acceptance of the demonstration by Medicare+Choice plans and limit HCFA's ability a) to measure the impact of competitive pricing and b) to generalize demonstration results to the entire Medicare program. (U.S. Department of Health and Human Services, Competitive Pricing Advisory Committee 1999)

Given the lack of statutory authority, however, CPAC felt it had to exclude FFS from the demonstration. The decision was one of the main reasons health plans gave for their opposition to the demonstration. The American Association of Health Plans (AAHP), in particular, claimed that the demonstration would be guilty of "tilting competition unfairly against private plans" if FFS were excluded (Ignagni, quoted in Weinstein 1999). That criticism undoubtedly will be raised again in response to the Obama proposal.

Despite the lack of a formal FFS bid, two features of the demonstration linked plan payments to FFS. First, historical FFS costs served as the basis for determining a budget-neutral cap on the government contribution to M+C premiums in the demonstration. Given that local area advisory committees (AACs) had specified a relatively generous benefits package, it was expected that M+C plans' bids for this package would be in the neighborhood of the cap. Thus, FFS costs would have some effect in constraining the bids by plans, although they would not directly affect premiums paid by FFS beneficiaries.

Premium Rebates. Second, low-bidding plans in the Denver demonstration were allowed to offer premium rebates. This option was added late in the design phase of the project. Premium rebates represented a very important link between FFS and the demonstration. A low-bidding M+C plan that offered a premium rebate could reduce its price below the Part B premium that FFS enrollees would pay for their coverage, thereby creating direct price competition between M+C plans and FFS. To be sure, this price competition came in the form of opportunities for reduced premiums for low-bidding M+C plans rather than increased premiums for FFS, as would follow from complete inclusion of FFS. But it appeared to be an answer to the vexing problem of including FFS in the competitive pricing system.

Feldman and others (2001) noted that premium rebates had become part of the "quiet consensus" for Medicare reform, and that they were included in a number of reform proposals at the time. In 2003, they were authorized for M+C plans. M+C plans now had the option of electing payment reductions of up to 125 percent of the Part B premium and returning 80 percent of the reduction—that is, up to the whole Part B premium—to beneficiaries in the form of a rebate. Apart from the "tax" on premium rebates, FFS might now appear to be included in the competitive pricing system by virtue of the ability of MA plans to create price differentials between themselves and FFS.

But is getting a rebate like paying a premium? In the current payment system, a low bidder gets to offer attractive optional benefits or premium rebates if it thinks these inducements will attract enrollees from FFS and other MA plans. In contrast, in a competitive bidding system that included FFS, a low bid would mean that competing plans—including FFS—would have to charge out-of-pocket (OOP) premiums above and beyond the Part B premium. To economists, carrots and sticks are equal. Receiving a premium rebate of $1 to join an MA plan or paying $1 to stay in FFS are equivalent options that create the same cash incentive of $1 to join the MA plan. Behavioral scientists, however, point to the results of laboratory experiments and some market evidence that disputes this equivalence (Borges and Knetsch 1997; Horowitz and McConnell 2003). In particular, people may have a tendency to value an object more if they own it and are offered money to part with it than if they don't own it and are offering money to acquire it. If these differences were large, and if people perceived a "right" to enroll in FFS Medicare at no more than the Part B premium, they might have to be paid more to give up this right than they would be willing to pay to keep it. In other words, rebates would have to be larger than OOP premiums to elicit the same behavioral response (plan-switching). Knowing this, plans would discount the effectiveness of premium rebates and, therefore, they would not be as likely to submit low bids in the current payment system as in a system that "truly" included FFS Medicare.

While an extended discussion is beyond the scope of this book, we have several reservations about the reported difference between willingness to pay for FFS Medicare and willingness to be paid to leave it. First, the largest differences have been found when people are asked how much they would have to be paid to give up irreplaceable public goods—such as permitting development in Yellowstone National Park (Hanemann 1991). This example does not seem like a good analogy for the choice among Medicare health plans. Second, the difference reported in a laboratory experiment can be biased if the experiment is poorly designed. For example, the difference tends to shrink as subjects gain more practice with reporting their valuations of willingness to pay and willingness to accept. In the most careful experimental study to date, Plott and Zeiler (2003) found no difference between willingness to pay and willingness to accept. Third, a profit-maximizing entrepreneur could make money by exploiting the difference between willingness to pay and willingness to accept (Hoffman and Spitzer 1993). Unless such "arbitrageurs" were banned, they could drive the difference to zero. Fourth, if people attached greater value to objects they hold than to those they might acquire, the result would be unusual or anomalous behavior. For instance, no one ever would sell a non-depreciating object for less than he or she paid for it; and Medicare health plans' prices would be "sticky"—that is, not likely to change even if costs changed exogenously by a large amount. This is a standard result from the "kinky" demand curve that would occur if consumer demand for MA plans were relatively elastic for price increases but inelastic for price decreases (Stigler 1947). Empirical evidence (Town and Liu 2003) is, however, inconsistent with the idea that MA plans' premiums are invariant to cost differences.

Finally, the (possible) difference between beneficiaries' willingness to accept rebates and their willingness to pay for FFS implies that our estimates of the savings from competitive pricing are *minimum* estimates. But the minimum estimates provide strong evidence that the savings would be substantial.

Bidding against Known versus Unknown Benchmarks. Our proposed bidding model differs from the current MA payment system in one significant way: In our proposal, the benchmark for determining the government payment would be set by all plans' bids, not by FFS costs alone; therefore, except for the FFS bid, it would be unknown to plans when they submitted their bids. In contrast, under the current payment system, plans know the FFS-based benchmark in advance of submitting bids. Would this difference create incentives for plans to submit higher or lower bids?

Theoretical models of bidding behavior do not provide a clear answer to this question. The canonical reading on the theory of a firm facing uncertain demand is Leland's 1972 article. According to Leland, if the firm's objective is profit-maximization, then uncertainty in the payment rate introduced by any type of bidding—whether against a known or unknown benchmark—would not affect its bid because only one bid maximizes expected profits. For uncertainty to make any difference in the bid, we have to assume that firms also care about the difference between expected and actual profits. Firms that maximize expected utility (rather than expected profit) would care about this difference, for example.

Next, we need to specify the penalties for bidding too high or too low *ex post*.[3] In both cases, profit will fall short of the expected maximum. But will a high bid be penalized more than a low one? This depends on whether Medicare MA plans have *economies* or *diseconomies* of scale. "Economy of scale" means that the average cost of enrollment falls as enrollment increases. This would be the case if MA plans had high fixed costs—such as the cost of setting up a provider network—but low marginal costs. If economies of scale are present, then low *ex post* bids will be penalized less than high bids because low bids bring in additional enrollment, which will reduce the plan's average cost. On the other hand, diseconomies of scale will penalize low bids more than high bids, and constant returns to scale will penalize low and high bids equally.

As noted in chapter 1, Wholey and colleagues (1996) found that local HMOs (the only type of MA plan for which such estimates are available) have large economies of scale up to about 6,000 Medicare enrollees and modest economies of scale up to at least 12,000 enrollees. Ruth Given (1996) also found economies of scale up to about 50,000 Medicare enrollees. There is no level of output in either study at which HMOs have diseconomies of scale for Medicare enrollment. Consequently, HMOs might feel that submitting low bids is less risky when they bid against an unknown benchmark, and this feeling may be stronger among small

HMOs. We will explore the implications of small HMOs submitting low bids when we discuss capacity constraint issues below.

Whatever economic theory predicts, Berenson argued that bidding against an unknown benchmark "creates different dynamics" than bidding against a known benchmark:

> Indeed, in their opposition to the competitive-pricing demon-strations, plans expressed concern that the added uncertainty provided by the lack of an external benchmark might lead them to make lower bids than they would otherwise make. Thus, in the MMA model, with all plans bidding against a known bench-mark, bids may cluster closer to the external benchmark than they would in the competitive pricing model. (Berenson 2004, w4-580)

John Cawley and Andrew Whitford (2007) raised an additional con-cern that the known benchmark could be used as a focal point for collusive bidding. They pointed out that in the initial round of bidding for regional PPOs in 2006, one region had an average plan bid exactly equal to the statutory benchmark.[4]

If Berenson is correct in thinking that bidding against an unknown benchmark changes the market dynamics, or if collusive bidding against a known benchmark is pervasive, bidding against an unknown benchmark, as in our competitive pricing proposal, apparently could result in lower average bids than bidding against a known benchmark.

How Should the Government Premium Contribution Be Set?

In the past, we have proposed that "Medicare's premium contribution should be set equal to the lowest price submitted by a qualified health plan in the market area" (Dowd, Feldman, and Christianson 1996, 158). The prices presumably would be submitted in sealed bids, as they were in the Denver demonstration.

Another way to set the government premium contribution, however, is to use the model of an auction, in which a seller wants to get the highest possible price for an object he owns. In this case, the buyer (Medicare) wants to purchase health plans' services for beneficiaries at the lowest possible price; but the logic is the same and is easily explained by a seller's auction. Would Medicare want to purchase health plans' services using the system we proposed?

Suppose the seller asked for sealed bids and announced that he would accept the highest one. A potential buyer who suspected that his valuation of the object was much higher than that of other bidders might be tempted to bid slightly less than his true value. This strategy would increase the risk of losing the object, but if his bid were successful it would increase his profit (the difference between his value and his bid). Thus, buyers in a "first-price, sealed-bid" auction tend to "shade" their bids downward (Dixit and Skeath 2004). Other things equal, sellers would prefer that buyers not shade their bids downward.

William Vickrey (1961) showed how to design an auction that promoted truthful revelation of buyers' valuations. Suppose buyers submitted sealed bids, with the highest bidder getting the object but at the second-highest bid. Now, bidders would submit truthful bids because doing so would increase their chances of getting the object but would not decrease their profits. Thus, a "second-price, sealed-bid auction" has been dubbed "Vickrey's truth serum" (Dixit and Skeath 2004).

The problem with Vickrey's truth serum is that buyers reveal their true valuations only because this gives them some profit, which reduces the seller's profit. Whether the seller makes more profit from the second-price auction than from the first-price auction is not clear. Suppose buyers are risk-averse, meaning they are much more concerned about the losses caused by underbidding (and not acquiring the object) than about the costs of bidding their true valuations. If so, we would expect them not to shade their bids very much, and the seller would earn more profit by holding a first-price auction than a second-price auction.

In the case of bidding for Medicare contracts, the costs of shading a bid upward are more complex than in the simple example of bidding for a single object, but they are likely to be quite large compared with the gains. Suppose the plan shades its bid upward but nevertheless is the low bidder. It would receive a larger government premium contribution and still be able to avoid charging an OOP premium. The plan's rivals, however, also would receive the larger premium contribution, given the higher level of the lowest bid. In other words, a winning bid-shader creates a positive externality for other plans, which it would not want to do (even though the *relative* position of plans is unaffected). Now suppose the bid-shader loses to another plan. All plans receive a higher premium contribution equal to the winning rival's bid, so there is still an externality (albeit smaller than before), and the bid-shader has to charge an OOP premium because it is not the lowest bidder. Therefore, bid-shading seems suboptimal whether the shading plan wins or loses. We doubt that holding a second-price, sealed-bid auction would save money for Medicare compared with our proposed first-price, sealed-bid auction.

Two problems that might arise when the government contribution is based on the lowest bid (or even the second-lowest bid) are, first, that the low bidder may not have adequate capacity to serve all beneficiaries who want to enroll, and, second, that the low bid may be an unreliable estimate of the cost of an efficient health plan in the local market area.

In the first instance, capacity constraints may be important because private plans know that a competitive pricing process will result in some plans being "free" (available for no more than the Part B premium), while others have to charge an OOP premium. But they do not know whether their bid will result in an OOP premium or how beneficiaries will respond to OOP premium differences. In the competitive pricing demonstrations authorized by the Balanced Budget Act of 1997, the HCFA decided to remove some of the uncertainty by allowing HMOs to set a maximum enrollment limit. The aim was to ensure an adequate supply to serve the local market area. If HMOs have economies of scale for Medicare enrollment, however, issues of enrollment uncertainty may be less important than the likelihood that small plans will submit low bids to increase their enrollment and benefit from economies of scale, as discussed above.

By "capacity constraints," we mean that MA plans' marginal costs rise rapidly after reaching a critical output where further expansion is constrained because the supply of a key resource is fixed. Given the evidence cited above that some HMOs have economies of scale for Medicare enrollment, it is unlikely that they face capacity constraints.[5]

The second problem with the lowest bid—that it may not be a reliable estimate of the cost of an efficient health plan in the local market area—could presumably occur if the low bidder is rash or inexperienced, especially if it is a new plan or one with low enrollment. Again, given the evidence that small plans have economies of scale and the inference that they will submit low bids, this problem is plausible. Is it likely, though? Given some basic monitoring of health plan quality, it is hard to see why the lowest-priced plan would be unpopular. Empirical evidence (Dowd, Feldman, and Coulam 2003; Atherly, Dowd, and Feldman 2004) suggests that Medicare beneficiaries gravitate toward, not away from, low prices. But the lowest-priced plan could, in various ways, be an inadequate product. Concerns could also arise over the legitimacy of the lowest bid. It might be predatory or simply too low to be realistic.[6] A plan that underestimated its costs, for example, might become the low bidder and thereby determine the government contribution. Yet, at that rate, this plan (and presumably others) would experience losses, with a possible effect on the quality of care.

If the legitimacy of the lowest bid is questionable, is there a role for the government to play in correcting this problem? Dowd and others (1996) proposed to place health plans with uncertain quality on probation before bids are collected. A probationary bidder could not be the low bidder that determined the government's premium contribution. If a probationary plan submitted the lowest bid, its contribution would be equal to the lowest nonprobationary bid. As a result, beneficiaries would be guaranteed access to the core benefit package from at least one nonprobationary plan for no more than the Part B premium.

Another possible response would be to evaluate plans' bids against an unannounced "minimum reasonable bid" and to base the government contribution on the lowest bid that exceeds the minimum reasonable bid. This strategy undercuts the basic premise behind competitive bidding, however—plans should tell the government what it costs to produce Medicare enrollment, and not the other way around. Having the government tell plans what is a reasonable bid would introduce administrative pricing into the bidding system. Plans would try to guess the minimum reasonable bid (which would be easy after observing the results of several rounds of bidding), and those with lower costs would submit bids equal to the minimum. Consequently, the government contribution would be set at an unnecessarily high level.

In summary, setting the government's contribution equal to the lowest bid from a qualified health plan is likely to save more money for Medicare than setting the contribution equal to the second-lowest bid. Concerns that the low bidder will have capacity constraints are unlikely to be justified. The CMS can address concerns that the lowest bid is unreliable or illegitimate by placing plans of uncertain quality on probationary status rather than attempting to assess the reasonableness of bids.

4

Estimating the Savings from Competitive Pricing in Medicare

Throughout this book, we have stressed that Medicare is in critical financial condition, and that something must be done to save money for the program. We have also noted that competitive pricing, while not the whole solution to this financial crisis, could be part of the solution. In this chapter, we review past estimates of the savings from the Medicare HMO program and from competitive pricing models that rely on bids from Medicare HMOs as well as fee-for-service (FFS) to set the government payment rate. Next, we calculate the likely savings from MedPAC's proposal to "level the playing field" by paying all plans at the level of FFS cost (U.S. Medicare Payment Advisory Commission 2007a; U.S. House of Representatives, Committee on the Budget 2007), and we compare these to estimates of the savings from several competitive pricing designs, including one recently proposed by the Obama administration that would exclude FFS Medicare. We find that MedPAC's proposal would save only a very small amount of money, as would an average-bid model that uses both FFS and private plans' bids to create a single weighted-average bid. The Obama administration's proposal is more effective but still would save only 1.79 percent of total Medicare spending. A competitive pricing model that uses the lower of the average private plan bid or the FFS bid to set the payment rate for all plans would save more money. The most effective system in terms of savings would use the lowest bid from any qualified plan (FFS or private) to set the payment rate for all Medicare health plans. In other words, any system using other than the lowest qualified bid would impose *enormous* extra costs.

Savings from the Medicare HMO Program

Efforts to estimate the savings from reduced use of resources by enrollees in Medicare HMOs date back to a 1993 study by Brown and others, which found that HMO enrollees spent over 10 percent less for Medicare-covered physician, hospital, home health, and skilled nursing facility (SNF) services than the amount they would have spent in traditional Medicare. Almost all of the savings resulted from a 17 percent reduction in hospital days among HMO enrollees.

HMO efficiencies would result in savings to the government if HMO bids were used to set the payment rate for Medicare health plans. The first published estimate of the savings from competitive pricing was provided by Thorpe and Atherly (2001), who estimated that competitive pricing with the government payment tied to the average Medicare+Choice plan bid in the beneficiary's county of residence would save $16 billion in 2002 (about 8 percent of total Medicare expenditures for the aged population), almost all due to higher payments by FFS beneficiaries to remain in FFS.

Next, in 2006, the Congressional Budget Office estimated that setting the government payment equal to the minimum bid in each county would have saved 8–11 percent of Medicare costs in 2004. Setting the payment equal to the enrollment-weighted average bid in each county would have reduced costs by only 1–2 percent. The CBO noted that these estimates were subject to "great uncertainty"[1] and assumed that per-capita spending in the traditional Medicare program would not be affected by competitive pricing (U.S. Congressional Budget Office 2006, 40n17).

Thorpe and Atherly's estimate of the savings from an average-bid payment system exceeded the CBO's estimate because they attributed greater efficiency to private plans, assuming the average M+C plan could provide standard Medicare benefits for 84 percent of what it cost traditional Medicare in fiscal year 2002. They based this cost differential on unpublished CBO data as well as the bids submitted by managed-care plans in the Denver demonstration site and reported by Dowd (2001). On the other hand, in published data, the CBO attributed an overall efficiency advantage of 3 percent to FFS in 2005, although private plans were 8 percent more efficient than FFS in the highest-cost counties (U.S. Congressional Budget Office 2006, table 2-1).

Thorpe and Atherly also calculated the average bid using only M+C plan bids, whereas the CBO included FFS Medicare in its calculation. The effect of this difference on the estimated savings from competitive pricing depends on whether FFS is less expensive, on average, than HMOs. Had the CBO excluded FFS from the average bid, its savings estimate would have been lower because of its assumption that FFS was less expensive than HMOs. Had Thorpe and Atherly included FFS, their savings estimate would have been lower because of their assumption that FFS was more expensive than HMOs.

We should also note that all of the models estimated to date, including our own, have been *static* models based on current data. None has included a *dynamic* effect of competition on the types of medical technology that are developed, the supply of physicians by specialty, the substitution of lower-cost medical personnel, changes in the provision of medically ineffective treatments, or a host of other possible effects. Because our model is a *static* model, we do not assume any compounding of the savings over time. This logic applies to all of our savings computations.

Estimates of Savings and Beneficiary Disruption

In this section, we estimate the savings from MedPAC's proposal and from several competitive pricing systems. Competitive bidding among all plans, with the payment rate set by the lowest bid from any qualified plan, will save more money for Medicare—by far—than any other payment system. This system is, however, the most disruptive to Medicare beneficiaries.

Savings Estimates. We use data from a variety of sources, but primarily MedPAC and the CBO, to estimate the savings from five payment systems:

- MedPAC's proposal to "level the playing field" by paying all plans at the level of FFS cost;

- a competitive pricing model that uses both FFS' and private plans' bids to create a single weighted-average bid;

- competitive bidding among all plans with the payment rate set by the lower of the average private plan bid or the FFS bid;

- competitive bidding among all plans with the payment rate set by the lowest bid from any qualified plan; and

- the Obama administration's proposal for bidding only among private (MA) plans.

Our savings estimates assume there would be no tax for bids below the benchmark: Plans bidding below the benchmark in all systems would receive the benchmark payment without the 25 percent tax presently paid by low-bidding plans.

The data for our calculations are shown in the upper panel of table 4-1 according to the level of FFS costs in 2005. Counties are grouped into FFS cost ranges of less than $550, $550–$599, $600–$649, $650–$699, and $700 or more. All costs are "per member per month" (PMPM) unless otherwise noted. The current benchmark for MA plan payments in each county cost range is shown in the second column. The benchmark in all counties is greater than FFS cost, and it is substantially greater in the low-cost counties. The next two columns show the fractions of Medicare beneficiaries and MA enrollees residing in each county cost range. This is followed by estimates of the minimum and average MA plan bids as a ratio of FFS costs. The minimum bid is equal to FFS costs in the lowest-cost counties, and the ratio falls as FFS costs increase. The ratio of average bids to FFS costs also decreases as FFS costs increase, but the average bids are higher than FFS costs until FFS costs reach approximately $650 PMPM. The message is that MA plans are less efficient than FFS in low-cost counties and more efficient than FFS in high-cost counties.

The results of our calculations are shown in the lower panel of table 4-1, starting with MedPAC's proposal. By tying MA plan payments to FFS costs, MedPAC's proposal would save $15.34 PMPM in the lowest-cost counties (data not shown). Because these counties have only 15 percent of all Medicare beneficiaries, however, those savings on a PMPM basis across all Medicare beneficiaries would be only $2.30 per month. The savings would decrease until they were negligible in the counties with the highest FFS costs. Overall, MedPAC's proposal would save $5.65 PMPM in 2005, or approximately 1 percent of Medicare costs ($2.9 billion).

Under the first "average-bid" model, a single weighted-average bid would be calculated from the FFS bid and private plans' bids. This system is similar to the CBO's average-bid model and is also the proposed approach for setting the benchmark in the 2010 CCA demonstration. Because FFS is the largest health plan (by enrollment) in most market areas, its bid would get the heaviest weight; consequently, this bidding model is very similar to MedPAC's proposal for paying all health plans at the FFS level. This similarity is reflected in the small savings estimate of $5.76 PMPM, only a few cents more than MedPAC's proposal. The annual savings to Medicare in 2005 would be $3 billion.

Under the second "average-bid" system, following Thorpe and Atherly (2001), the government payment rate would be equal to the lower of the FFS bid or the average MA plan bid. The results for counties with low and medium FFS costs would be identical to MedPAC's proposal because FFS Medicare is the lowest bidder in those counties, containing over half of all MA enrollees. The average MA plan bid would be higher than the FFS bid until FFS costs reached $650 or more. The largest savings of $15.96 PMPM would be found in counties where FFS costs exceeded $700. Overall, this proposal would save $25.57 PMPM in 2005, or approximately 4 percent of Medicare costs ($13.1 billion).

Under the "minimum-bid" system, Medicare expenditures would fall in all counties except those with the lowest FFS costs. As in the average-bid systems (especially the second one), the savings would increase in areas with higher FFS costs. Overall, basing the government payment to all Medicare health plans on the minimum bid submitted by any qualified plan would save $52.73 PMPM in 2005, or approximately 8 percent of Medicare costs ($27.1 billion).

On February 26, 2009, the Obama administration released its proposed federal budget for 2010 (U.S. Office of Management and Budget 2009). To make a "down payment" on fundamental reform of the health-care system, the president proposed to create a $630 billion fund over ten years. Approximately 28 percent of that fund, $177 billion over ten years, would come from a competitive bidding program for Medicare Advantage plans, starting in 2012. While some details of the program were not spelled out, observers expected it to "slash payments to private insurers" (Fuhrmans 2009). But would it save much money for Medicare?

TABLE 4-1

MEDICARE SAVINGS FROM MEDPAC AND COMPETITIVE BIDDING PROPOSALS

A. RELATION OF BID TO FFS COSTS, BY COUNTY FFS COST RANGE

FFS cost range	Current benchmark	Fraction of Medicare beneficiaries	Fraction of MA enrollees	Minimum bid/FFS cost*	Average bid/FFS cost**
<$550	$684	0.150	0.142	1.00	1.16
$550–$599	$655	0.201	0.201	0.98	1.05
$600–$649	$681	0.235	0.234	0.94	1.01
$650–$699	$711	0.152	0.153	0.92	0.96
$700+	$777	0.263	0.270	0.86	0.92

B. TOTAL SAVINGS PMPM FOR COUNTIES IN EACH FFS COST RANGE

FFS cost range	Savings estimates (PMPM)			
	MedPAC	Average bid (1)	Average bid (2)	Minimum bid
<$550	$2.30	$0.76	$2.30	$2.30
$550–$599	$1.70	$0.97	$1.70	$4.01
$600–$649	$1.16	$0.98	$1.16	$10.04
$650–$699	$0.31	$0.84	$4.45	$8.58
$700+	$0.18	$2.21	$15.96	$27.80
Total PMPM	**$5.65**	**$5.76**	**$25.57**	**$52.73**

SOURCES: U.S. House of Representatives, Committee on the Budget 2007; U.S. Congressional Budget Office 2006; U.S. Department of Health and Human Services, Centers for Medicare and Medicaid Services n.d.b.; and U.S. Boards of Trustees 2008.
NOTES: * = Ratio of estimated minimum bid to FFS cost; ** = Ratio of average bid to FFS cost; Med-PAC = Benchmark set at FFS cost; Average bid (1) = Benchmark set at weighted average of FFS and MA bids; Average bid (2) = Benchmark set at lower of FFS bids or weighted-average MA bid; Minimum bid = Benchmark set at lowest bid of a qualified plan.

The most important detail to be spelled out is whether the competitive bidding program would include all Medicare health plans or just private MA plans. Based on a statement by Peter Orszag, director of the Office of Management and Budget, including FFS Medicare at this time would be "unhelpful," and it is more important to focus on efforts to improve the efficiency of

TABLE 4-2

MEDICARE SAVINGS FROM COMPETITIVE BIDDING FOR MA PLANS ONLY

FFS cost range	% of MA enrollees	Low MA plan bid	Savings per member per month	Total savings (2005)
<$550	0.142	$540.00	$129.26	$1,182,029,703
$550–$599	0.201	$563.50	$78.86	$1,020,810,772
$600–$649	0.234	$592.20	$77.39	$1,166,259,327
$650–$699	0.153	$625.60	$70.78	$697,420,956
$700+	0.27	$645.00	$110.33	$1,918,423,330
Total				$5,984,944,088

SOURCE: Authors' calculations.

FFS Medicare (Orszag 2009). So we interpret the Obama proposal as an MA-only bidding system.

We simulated the likely savings from an "MA-only" bidding system that uses the most effective design for reducing payments to MA plans: setting the government contribution equal to the minimum bid submitted by any MA plan in the local area. The results are shown in table 4-2. The annual savings from MA-only competitive bidding would have been almost $6 billion in 2005, or 1.79 percent of total Medicare spending in that year. The largest proportion of the savings, about one-third, would have come from areas with the highest FFS cost, in which 27 percent of MA enrollment is found. While this estimate is larger than the 1 percent savings from Med-PAC's proposal or from a bidding system that uses the weighted average of all bids to pay all plans, it is much smaller than the 8 percent savings from using the lowest bid to pay all plans.

These estimates are sensitive to changing levels of MA plan enrollment, which have risen since 2005. Any growth in MA enrollment would enhance the effectiveness of an MA-only bidding system, though it seems unlikely that MA enrollment would grow under such a system in which MA plans bid on the entitlement benefit package. Also, the savings estimates could be different if Congress were to change MA payment rates by legislation.

Notwithstanding these caveats, it appears that exempting FFS from competitive bidding would not harness the power of efficient health plans to reduce Medicare costs.

These results also help explain why the CCA demonstration required by the Medicare Modernization Act of 2003 will save only a very small amount of money, which we estimate to be about 1 percent of total Medicare costs. The reason for this low estimate is that the CCA uses a single weighted-average bid, which will be driven by the FFS bid in most areas. As a result, MA enrollees in areas with low FFS costs will pay higher out-of-pocket premiums, but the overall savings will be small because they come almost entirely from reduced payments to MA plans. In addition, because the CCA bidding model is driven by the FFS bid, it closely resembles MedPAC's proposal—which, we have pointed out, represents a return to the AAPCC.

Beneficiary Disruption. Next we estimate the degree of beneficiary disruption that could result from various bidding models, expressing it in terms of dollar values. For some beneficiaries, the dollars are out-of-pocket premiums they would have to pay for the entitlement benefit package from FFS Medicare in areas where FFS is a high bidder. For others, the dollars represent out-of-pocket premiums they would have to pay to continue receiving nonentitlement benefits they used to receive for free from an MA plan.

It is crucial to distinguish among three sources of disruption in our proposal. First, our proposal removes the "floor" payments in counties with low FFS Medicare costs. Second, our proposal reduces the government's payment to all health plans to the level of the lowest bid by a qualified health plan in each county *for the entitlement benefit package*, which means that all additional benefits are paid for out of pocket. This form of disruption affects current MA enrollees only. Third, our proposal subjects FFS Medicare to direct price competition with private plans.

Other payment options are more limited in the ways they cause disruption. MedPAC's proposal creates the first type of disruption. The Obama administration's proposal creates the first and second types.

Our disruption analysis assumes no changes in enrollments will follow changes in out-of-pocket premiums under competitive bidding models compared with the status quo. This means that our estimates represent the maximum amount of disruption experienced by beneficiaries who stay in their previous plans. Some beneficiaries will decide the extra premium is not worth it and will switch to less expensive alternatives that may be "almost as good" as their current choice. Others will have to disenroll to different plans when their current plan exits the market; their new choice (albeit forced) could be almost as good as the current one. Despite the ability to mitigate it by switching plans, we note that this type of disruption figured prominently in the opposition of local areas to hosting a demonstration of competitive bidding (U.S. Department of Health and Human Services, Competitive Pricing Advisory Commission 2001). Medicare beneficiaries can be a powerful force to block demonstrations when they have to pay higher premiums.

Changes in an average beneficiary's monthly out-of-pocket premium under each bidding model are shown in table 4-3.[2] This table gives us a picture of who would be financially disrupted and how much they would be disrupted under each bidding model. Under MedPAC's proposal, FFS beneficiaries would not be disrupted at all because the government contribution is equal to FFS costs in all areas. All MA enrollees would be disrupted, however, because MedPAC's proposal would reduce MA plan payments in all areas of the country, especially those with low FFS costs.

The first average-bid model is the only one in which some beneficiaries would be better off compared with the status quo. (Negative numbers = better off, as shown in parentheses.) These fortunate individuals are FFS beneficiaries in areas with low FFS costs, and their good fortune would be due to high MA bids in those areas that raised the weighted-average bid for all plans, including FFS, resulting in premium rebates to FFS enrollees.[3] MA enrollees in areas with low FFS costs would pay substantially higher premiums under both average-bid models.

Under the second average-bid model, FFS beneficiaries in lowest cost areas would not be disrupted because FFS would be the winning bidder in those areas. MA enrollees would be disrupted in all areas of the country— even those where their bids are lower than FFS costs on average. This would occur because MA plan payments in those areas currently are greater than their bids.

The most disruption would occur under the minimum-bid model. FFS beneficiaries would be disrupted because the MA sector's minimum bid would set the payment rate in all areas except those with very low FFS

TABLE 4-3

DISRUPTION ($PMPM) FOR AVERAGE FFS AND MA ENROLLEE IN EACH FFS COST RANGE

FFS cost range	—MedPAC—		—Average bid (1)—		—Average bid (2)—	
	FFS	MA	FFS	MA	FFS	MA
<$550	$ –	($129.26)	$10.26	($119.00)	$ –	($129.26)
$550–$599	$ –	($67.36)	$3.61	($63.76)	$ –	($67.36)
$600–$649	$ –	($39.59)	$0.79	($38.81)	$ –	($39.59)
$650–$699	$ –	($16.38)	($0.43)	($19.82)	($27.20)	($43.58)
$700+	$ –	($5.33)	($7.72)	($13.06)	($60.00)	($65.33)

FFS cost	————Minimum bid————	
	FFS	MA
<$550	$ –	($129.26)
$550–$599	($11.50)	($78.86)
$600–$649	($37.80)	($77.39)
$650–$699	($54.40)	($70.78)
$700+	($105.00)	($110.33)

SOURCE: Authors' calculations.
NOTE: Negative numbers = worse off = disruption; positive numbers = better off.

costs. MA enrollees would be disrupted because the minimum bids would be lower than the amounts that HMOs currently are paid.

To summarize these calculations: MedPAC's proposal would hit MA enrollees in areas with low FFS costs hardest; the average-bid models would hit all MA enrollees and FFS beneficiaries in areas with high FFS costs; and the low-bid model would hit almost everyone. For some purposes, this rank ordering of impacts is a rank ordering of political difficulty, which we discuss later.

Special attention must be paid to the effects of any reform proposal on lower-income beneficiaries who do not qualify for Medicaid. In areas of high FFS costs, those beneficiaries would be affected by the minimum-bid proposal in two ways: Premiums for FFS Medicare could increase dramatically, and drug coverage from MA plans would no longer be low-cost or free. We know that MA enrollees are disproportionately minority or low-income beneficiaries (Thorpe and Atherly 2002), so at face value, that kind of disruption seems unfair. Overpaying MA plans for the entitlement benefit package, however, is a notably unfair and inefficient way to provide assistance to lower-income beneficiaries. Why should only low-income beneficiaries in areas with high FFS costs receive that kind of assistance with supplementary benefits? Since this assistance to *some* lower-income beneficiaries just happens to fall out of large overpayments, how do we know this is the right amount of assistance? We should not glorify low-income subsidies that derive from what, in fact, are simply overpayments from a bad system. And why should the wealthy in those high-payment areas receive any assistance at all? The Part D Low Income Subsidy (LIS) program is a better model of how to provide additional help to lower-income beneficiaries. Another option for providing such assistance would be an income-related credit or voucher to purchase insurance of any kind. Both options would provide appropriate subsidies for low-income beneficiaries, while letting Medicare address the problem of getting its payments right.

5

Should FFS Medicare Be Allowed Greater Flexibility?

If the government contribution to the premiums of both FFS and private plans were based on the lowest bid by a qualified health plan, current data suggest that FFS Medicare would be the lower-cost plan in some market areas, while private plans would be lower-cost in other areas. Those data are, however, based on the current benefit designs and organizational structures of both FFS Medicare and private plans. Greater price competition might lead private plans to change their benefits or organizational structure, and, except for the mandate to cover the entitlement benefit package, private plans have the freedom to make those changes. Obvious questions arise: Should FFS Medicare be given the same flexibility? What types of flexibility might be involved?

Opinions regarding the degree to which FFS Medicare should be allowed greater flexibility will depend on how one views the necessity of having an FFS plan in Medicare. Our stated purposes of Medicare do not identify an exclusive role for either public or private plans and certainly no unique role for a health plan that happens to pay its providers on an FFS basis, as opposed to capitation or salary. We have argued that both types of plans have advantages and disadvantages. But others may feel differently. If one believes it is necessary for Medicare to offer all beneficiaries a plan that does not exclude "any willing providers" on the basis of their costs, then there would be no point to allowing FFS Medicare the freedom to offer, for example, a "preferred provider" plan that did exactly that.

Our position is that the FFS Medicare should do no more and no less than any other Medicare health plan: It should offer beneficiaries the features for which they are willing to pay, subject to offering the entitlement benefit package. We view that entitlement benefit in terms of health services that are covered, not in terms of the system in which they are delivered.

Congress specifies the entitlement benefit package for the Medicare program, but in chapter 1, we pointed out that Congress does not require the same benefit package of all health plans. Private plans, for example, are not required to contract with every provider that is willing to accept the FFS Medicare fee schedule, nor are they required to offer coverage in every part of the United States (though some private plans now do so). We concluded that these two benefits—open access and national service area—are not essential to carrying out the purposes of the Medicare program and, thus, should not be considered part of a comprehensive entitlement that applies to all beneficiaries. Instead, they represent a supplementary benefit that Congress desires FFS Medicare to offer, just as free health club memberships are a supplementary benefit that some private health plans desire to offer to their enrollees. It is perfectly reasonable for any health plan, including FFS Medicare or private health plans, to offer any supplementary benefit it likes; but when the government sets its contribution to premiums, it should be indifferent to the offering of these nonessential supplementary benefits. Plans should base their bids on the essential entitlement benefit package required of all health plans, and beneficiaries should pay the marginal cost of nonessential supplementary benefits out of their own pockets.

The following discussion evaluates several specific ways in which FFS Medicare might be granted greater flexibility. This topic could be interpreted as a discussion of leveling the playing field between FFS Medicare and private plans, and it is, to some extent. At the end of this section, however, we take up the broader topic of the level playing field and enumerate conditions that currently are imposed only on private plans. To have a truly level playing field, those conditions would need to be either dropped or imposed on FFS Medicare.

What Should FFS Medicare Be Allowed To Do?

The discussion of FFS flexibility will be facilitated by describing two types of initiatives that any rational health plan might undertake. Minimally, we expect any rational health plan to undertake any activity, including covering any service, that saves more than a dollar for each dollar spent. We refer to these as "cost-saving" initiatives.

Beyond cost-saving initiatives, we expect any rational health plan to offer any service for which its enrollees are willing to pay. These services would be cost-increasing, but they would be worth more than a dollar to enrollees for each dollar spent.

We want to see the entire Medicare menu of public and private health plans managed more efficiently. We favor head-to-head competition between FFS Medicare and private plans, and, in that environment, we believe that FFS Medicare should not be handicapped, but should be allowed the flexibility to compete effectively with private plans in the following ways.

Cover additional services. It is obvious to us that FFS Medicare should be allowed to make cost-saving coverage decisions. FFS should also be able to offer additional services (beyond the entitlement) if beneficiaries are willing to pay the cost of those services. Because they are not part of the entitlement, however, their marginal cost should be paid in full by beneficiaries. The precedent for such coverage is Medicare supplementary, or "Medigap," policies sold by private insurers, although as currently structured those policies are subject to a severe price distortion discussed in the section on "one-stop shopping," below. Medicare beneficiaries' preferences for supplementary coverage vary.[1] Several categories of standard Medicare supplementary policies accommodate such variation in preferences. Essentially, allowing FFS Medicare this new degree of flexibility would be equivalent to allowing it to sell its own supplementary insurance coverage.

Currently, outpatient prescription drug coverage and supplementary (Medigap) insurance are sold only by private plans and not by FFS Medicare. Not allowing FFS Medicare to sell its own Part D plans was one of the most controversial parts of the 2003 MMA legislation. This topic also is discussed in greater detail under "one-stop shopping."

Invest in administrative improvements. The same rules that apply to coverage also apply to investments in administrative improvements. If a particular administrative initiative has a positive return on investment and does not raise other issues (such as violating the purposes of Medicare), then FFS

Medicare should be able to make such an investment. If necessary, Congress could ask the CMS to submit a budget earmarked for such administrative investments and commission an independent audit of the actual return.

The more difficult issue concerns investments in administrative improvements that are not cost-saving, but for which beneficiaries are willing to pay. The example cited earlier was higher capacity to handle telephone or Internet inquiries from beneficiaries. Increased capacity would not save FFS Medicare money, but beneficiaries might be willing to pay for it. One technical difficulty is in making sure that beneficiaries, rather than non-Medicare-eligible taxpayers, *actually* pay for those administrative improvements. One way to do that would be to build their cost into the Part B premium. Another approach that might work in some cases would be to finance them through user fees, rather than through general assessments on all beneficiaries.

Offer an alternative plan. One of the principal differences between FFS Medicare and MA plans is in the area of provider contracting. MA plans must assure the Medicare program of their ability to provide adequate access to care for their enrollees. No such requirement is imposed on FFS Medicare. Within that constraint, however, MA plans have considerable freedom to develop their provider networks. Among a set of otherwise equally qualified providers, MA plans can select network providers on the basis of price and quality (for example, contracting only with those who can submit data from electronic health records) and reject providers who do not meet their standards. FFS Medicare currently does not have that degree of flexibility. It must contract with any provider who meets basic quality criteria and is willing to abide by the program's payment rules.

It would be reasonable to let FFS Medicare offer an alternative plan that features selective provider contracting based on the price and quality of providers. Furthermore, because open access to providers has been rejected by both the commercial insurance market and many low-income Medicare beneficiaries through their choice of MA plans with restricted networks, we conclude that open access is a supplementary benefit, and that beneficiaries who want that feature should purchase it out of pocket rather than with subsidies from taxpayers. In other words, the government should be allowed to offer a restricted-access plan and to base its bid in a competitive pricing system on the cost of that plan, rather than the optional open-access plan. Beneficiaries would pay the premium difference between the restricted-access plan and the open-access plan out of pocket.

If beneficiaries are willing to pay the marginal cost of open access out of their own pockets, then an open-access version of FFS Medicare will thrive. If not, then the open-access version will need to make other adjustments to its plan design, or hope that other advantages (such as monopsony pricing power, discussed in chapter 1) offset the higher premiums that open access implies. The same logic holds for any other constraint imposed only on FFS Medicare by Congress.

One model of restricted provider networks that retains freedom of choice is the preferred provider organization (PPO). Medicare has attempted to demonstrate PPOs, but the widespread purchase of supplementary insurance has been an important barrier to these demonstrations. Supplementary insurance generally covers the beneficiary's out-of-pocket costs, thereby reducing or eliminating any out-of-pocket price differences between preferred and nonpreferred providers.

The general difficulty with supplementary insurance is that the enrollee's total expenditures increase when the supplementary policy eliminates the effect of coinsurance and deductibles, and Medicare typically pays for about 80 percent of that increased utilization, while the supplementary insurer pays for the remaining 20 percent. This implicit price subsidy of private supplementary insurance resulting from the spillover effect of supplementary insurance on the Medicare program's budget has been recognized for at least twenty years (Christensen, Long, and Rodgers 1987), but Congress has taken no action to reduce it.

The situation with PPOs and supplementary insurance is a bit different, however. If the supplementary policy covered only the out-of-pocket costs of using nonpreferred providers, and Medicare's coverage of those costs were, say, 50 percent, rather than 80 percent, then the effect of the spillover problem would be proportionately reduced. The incentive to use preferred providers, however, would also be proportionately reduced, and convincing them to accept fee discounts in return for being on the preferred list would be more difficult.

The FFS PPO option would be most effective if its enrollees were prohibited from purchasing supplementary coverage, whether privately or through an employer. Alternatively, FFS Medicare could apply a tax to such policies to cover the spillover cost. The political barriers to either solution would be substantial, but consumers enrolled in PPOs in the commercial health insurance sector seem to fare quite well without supplementary policies.

Disease management. To provide the best possible care to its beneficiaries, FFS Medicare should be given the same flexibility as HMOs to install disease-management programs and incentives for providers to adhere to practice guidelines. Disease management could be a feature of a new, lower-cost FFS Medicare option. The unmanaged option could be retained for beneficiaries who prefer it—perhaps because they view disease-management as a form of rationing. Given how common disease management programs are for both MA plans and for the commercial market, "freedom from disease management" arguably is not an essential feature of Medicare. Thus, as in the case of open access, FFS Medicare's "bid" should be based on the cost of caring for beneficiaries in a plan that uses disease management, if it is demonstrated to reduce costs.

Offer one-stop shopping for Part D and supplementary coverage. MA enrollees can purchase basic Medicare coverage, coverage of outpatient prescription drugs, and any supplementary coverage they choose from a single health plan. FFS Medicare is prohibited from offering Part D coverage and supplementary insurance. Should FFS Medicare be able to sell those types of coverage? We answer that question by examining whether a "one-stop shopping" FFS Medicare product would correct any existing source of market failure and, if so, at what cost.

Allowing FFS Medicare to offer a one-stop shopping product might address a problem of restricted entry. If beneficiaries want the product, but it is currently unavailable in the market, then letting FFS Medicare sell Part D and supplementary coverage would increase efficiency.

Allowing FFS Medicare to offer supplementary coverage might also help address an important price distortion in Medicare. When beneficiaries purchase private supplementary insurance that covers their coinsurance and deductibles, the decrease in the point-of-purchase price of care results in increased demand for care (Atherly 2002). As mentioned above, about 80 percent of that additional cost is borne by FFS Medicare, while only

20 percent is built into the supplementary insurer's premium. As a result of this subsidy for the premiums of supplementary insurance policies, beneficiaries purchase inefficiently high levels of supplementary coverage and of health care. In theory, FFS Medicare could offer the supplementary coverage and price it correctly to eliminate the subsidy, but no one would buy that policy unless the same requirement were placed on sellers of private supplementary policies through a tax on supplementary insurance premiums. As noted earlier, Congress has not addressed the problem of public subsidies for private supplementary policies during the last twenty years, and thus we are not optimistic about this rationale for allowing FFS Medicare to sell supplementary insurance.

Allowing FFS Medicare to offer Part D coverage also is controversial, but for different reasons. If FFS Medicare were to offer its own Part D policy, it would almost certainly negotiate drug prices directly with pharmaceutical manufacturers—the prohibition of which was one of the most controversial parts of the 2003 MMA legislation. The final legislation denied FFS Medicare that option, even though, in theory, the government's prices could have been passed along to private Part D insurers.[2]

Some of the opposition to offering a public Part D plan may have been an attempt to protect drug company profits. Other opponents may have been concerned about further expansion of the public Medicare plan. A legitimate concern is the threat of inefficient monopsony pricing power on the part of the public plan, as discussed earlier. Approximately 80 percent of Medicare beneficiaries are in FFS Medicare, and if they all were to obtain their Part D coverage through a public plan, that plan would have enormous bargaining power with drug companies. Advocates of single-payer systems see the government's bulk purchasing power as an advantage, pointing to health systems in other countries that have not hesitated to exercise their market power. Opponents are concerned that the government might drive drug prices too low, resulting in reduced supply of existing drugs in the short run and suboptimal investment in the development of new drugs in the long run.[3]

Finally, we note the current debate over establishing a public health plan for the commercial health insurance sector. Part D generally is considered a successful program, and it does not include a public competitor for the private-sector plans. Whether those two facts are linked will undoubtedly be an important part of the broader health-care reform debate.

What Should Be Required of FFS Medicare?

Our discussion could leave the reader with the impression that all the imbalances in the current Medicare program force added costs on FFS Medicare that MA plans can avoid. There are two important exceptions, however. The first is the requirement that MA plans report HEDIS quality-of-care measures. The second is the requirement that MA plans provide adequate access to providers throughout their service areas.[4] FFS Medicare is not subject to either requirement. If Congress believes that both requirements are legitimate qualifications for any health plan to participate in the Medicare program, it should impose these requirements to an equal degree on FFS Medicare.

6

The Uneasy Relationship of Competitive Bidding to the Law and Politics of Medicare

In preceding chapters, we have provided a detailed justification for competitive pricing. But that justification generally has ignored a conspicuous historical reality. Anyone even dimly aware of Medicare's efforts to establish competitive bidding over the past decades knows that those efforts have been fraught with conflict and intense opposition. Not surprisingly, most policy analysts and policymakers now define the boundaries of "practical" or "achievable" reforms for Medicare well short of the comprehensive competitive pricing system we propose. As the *New York Times* noted when the comparative cost adjustment demonstration was included in the Medicare Modernization Act of 2003,

> Similar plans [to the CCA] have failed to find support among patients, doctors and hospitals, or even some insurers. Even people who favor the idea say the potential for trouble this time is formidable. "There is really no political constituency for competition," said Robert D. Reischauer, a health policy expert and a former director of the Congressional Budget Office. (Freudenheim 2003)

In view of this history of legal and political opposition, why do we nonetheless propose a comprehensive plan for competitive pricing? In this chapter, we address this troubled history to make a case why competitive pricing, including both public and private plans, should be considered.

Medicare's Attempts to Implement Competitive Pricing

Medicare has attempted to implement competitive pricing almost continuously since the program was established. Table 6-1 summarizes the most important efforts of the last twenty-five years. During that period, there have been at least eleven identifiable competitive pricing efforts. (Admittedly, the criteria here are somewhat subjective.) Given that these are multiyear projects in research, design, consultation, and implementation, it is fair to say that while there have been periods of more and less intense activity, competitive pricing efforts have been a fairly constant preoccupation of the HCFA and, later, the CMS.

The concerns from which these competitive pricing efforts arose go back to the very beginning of the Medicare program, when providers sought successfully to limit the government's exercise of its buying power. Note the following report from the U.S. General Accounting Office (1972, 3):

> Under the Medicare law [the Department of Health, Education, and Welfare] or its carriers are not allowed to negotiate with suppliers to secure lower prices for durable medical equipment.
>
> Such equipment is purchased by the Veterans Administration (VA), the Public Health Service, and a State Medicaid agency at discounted prices—often considerably less than the suppliers' list prices which are the basis for charges to Medicare. VA prices are specified in contracts which usually are awarded on the basis of competitive bids. . . . For example:
>
> - A supplier's Medicare price for a standard wheelchair was $122. The price for the same wheelchair under the VA contract was about $86, or 30 percent less.
>
> - A supplier's Medicare price for a hospital bed having safety sides was $336. The same bed under the VA contract was $270, or 20 percent, less.

This thirty-seven-year-old text is little different in substance from a report we could write today to describe all but one effort to introduce competitive

TABLE 6-1

PAST COMPETITIVE PRICING ATTEMPTS AND THEIR FATES
(IN ALPHABETICAL ORDER BY MEDICARE BENEFIT)

Period	Demonstration	Description
1991–96	Coronary artery bypass graft (CABG) demonstration	Negotiated bundled payment for Part A and B services for CABG, which allowed participating organizations to create payment approaches that rewarded physicians for reducing the cost of care.
1991–96	Cataract surgery alternate payment demonstration	Negotiated bundled payment for Part A and B services for cataract surgery.
Mid-1980s–87	Clinical laboratory services demonstration	Contractor-supported research and design effort, in preparation for implementation of demonstration.
Mid-1990s–2008	Clinical laboratory services demonstration.	Contractor-supported research and design effort required by the MMA. Demonstration designed, San Diego area selected.
Late 1980s	Durable medical equipment (DME) demonstration	Contractor-supported research and design effort, in preparation for implementation of demonstration.
Mid-1990s–2008	DME competitive bidding demonstration and subsequent nationwide implementation	Balanced Budget Act of 1997 authorized projects of competitive procurement of Medicare Part B services and items. Contractor-supported research and design effort, in preparation for implementation, with demonstration focused on selected high-volume items.

Results

The HCFA implemented the demonstration initially at four sites in three cities. Three other sites were later added. Pressure from providers significantly diluted the negotiation model—in the end, the model was reduced to a discounted bundle of Part A and B services. The CMS estimated the demonstration saved Medicare nearly $40 million (10 percent) in ten thousand CABGs performed at seven sites. The HCFA planned to expand the bypass demonstration project in March 1996; however, due to budget constraints caused by Y2K issues and the Balanced Budget Act of 1997, it put the project on hold. The demonstration gave rise to the "Centers of Excellence" program, based on "virtual bundling" within FFS payments.[1]

The ophthalmic community exerted constant pressure during the design of the demonstration, which led to the elimination of most of the demonstration's competitive features. Peer pressure among providers and a local boycott reduced participation. The ophthalmological society at one site (Cleveland) and the American Academy of Ophthalmology (AAO) sued to stop the demonstration, claiming it was beyond the government's authority and violated the ophthalmic community's rights to equal protection. After a year of deliberations and appeals, the ophthalmologists lost their lawsuit, but the suit hampered the demonstration. The HCFA ultimately implemented the demonstration at four sites in three cities. The CMS estimated that the demonstration resulted in modest savings to Medicare: more than $500,000 for some seven thousand surgeries.[2]

Under pressure from the clinical laboratory industry, Congress imposed a multiyear moratorium on competitive pricing activities for lab services in 1987.[3]

The clinical laboratory industry opposed the demonstration and sued to stop it. A federal judge in California granted a preliminary injunction prohibiting the CMS from announcing "winners" of bidding and carrying out the demonstration. Congress then repealed the CMS's authority to conduct a competitive bidding demonstration.[4]

Under pressure from the DME industry, Congress barred funds for the demonstration and substituted a fee schedule.[5]

Tested in Florida and Texas sites, the demonstration showed savings of 20 percent with no notable beneficiary harms.[6] The demonstration got this far mainly because a Florida senator and the Florida governor were notably active supporters of competitive bidding, and industry efforts to obtain injunctions in court were unsuccessful.[7] These demonstrations almost resulted in implementation program-wide. The expansion of the DME bidding program was set forth in the 2003 MMA, which required a phased introduction of competitive bidding for the ten largest metropolitan statistical areas (MSAs) in 2007, eighty of the largest MSAs in 2009, and additional areas after 2009. Providers were qualified according to enhanced quality

(continued on the next page)

(Table 6-1, continued from the previous page)

Period	Demonstration	Description
1995–97	Medicare HMO demonstration	Contractor-supported research and design work. Attempts to implement in Baltimore and Denver.
1997–2000	Medicare HMO demonstration	Contractor-supported research and design work, along with national and local expert panels required by BBA. Attempts to implement in Kansas City and Phoenix.
2010?	Medicare competitive cost adjustment demonstration	Competitive bidding for HMOs and FFS, scheduled to occur in 2010.
2006–8	Part B Competitive Acquisition Program (CAP) for drugs/biologicals	Contractor-supported research and design work. Vendors selected through bidding process to supply drugs to doctors and handle billing.
2006 and continuing	Part D payment system	Government payment amount based on the national average of plans' bids. Enrollee premiums reflect difference between each plan's bid and the nationwide average of plan bids.

SOURCE: Authors' research.

Results

requirements, and bids were received and evaluated for the first phase of this rollout. In 2008, the federal district court in the District of Columbia refused requests for a preliminary injunction.[8] But under pressure from industry, Congress delayed the program for eighteen months, thus giving time for a new round of lobbying to kill the program entirely.[9] The American Association for Homecare agreed in return to accept an almost 10 percent cut in fees for the items that were to be subject to bid—Congress required the quid pro quo because the program would cost more without competitive bidding.[10]

Congress stopped the Baltimore demonstration at the behest of city and state political leaders, under pressure from health plans and the local medical establishment, supported by some advocacy groups. The U.S. District Court issued a temporary restraining order to stop the Denver demonstration in a lawsuit brought by the American Association of Health Plans.[11] Bids that were submitted and examined showed savings of 25–38 percent compared with the government's payments to plans at that time. Congress then stopped the demonstration for reasons similar to those in Baltimore.[12]

Congress stopped the demonstration at the behest of city and state political leaders in Arizona, Kansas, and Missouri, under pressure from plans and the local medical establishment, supported by some advocacy groups.[13]

The CMS has yet to solicit contractor support to design the demonstration. Amendments have been introduced in Congress to kill the demonstration before it begins. No one of note predicts that the demonstration will actually occur, largely due to HMO opposition and rhetoric about beneficiary harm.

The MMA of 2003 required the implementation of the CAP for Part B drugs. In late 2005, the CMS conducted the first round of bidding for approved CAP vendors from whom participating physicians could obtain Part B drugs. The CAP was implemented in July 2006. Two years later, the CMS accepted bids for vendor contracts for the 2009–11 CAP. While the CMS received several qualified bids, contractual issues arose with the successful bidders (related to proprietary data). The CMS postponed the 2009 program indefinitely in September 2008.[14]

The bidding system was implemented in two years and has been successful in setting payments and premiums for Part D since 2006, with little complaint about the fact that it is "competitive pricing."

pricing for Medicare services. The policy argument against current administrative pricing methods remains as strong as it was almost four decades ago. All competitive pricing attempts *for existing Medicare benefits, with existing administrative pricing arrangements in place*, have failed in one critical sense: They have not replaced those administrative pricing mechanisms with competitive pricing mechanisms beyond the terms of the demonstration projects. These results have occurred despite the fact that all of the competitive demonstrations that reached the point of bid evaluation—even using bidding models that were frequently watered down under health plan or provider pressure—have demonstrated that they would save substantial amounts of money.

There is an exception to this record of failures: the successful introduction of competitive pricing for the Part D prescription drug benefit. That exception deserves separate comment.

The Exception: Competitive Pricing for a New Part D Benefit

When the MMA was passed in 2003, it established a voluntary prescription drug benefit. The benefit was to be provided by private plans only—that is, there would be no public plan, as in parts A and B.[15] Plans submit bids annually, based on their expected benefit payments for a beneficiary in average health. The government payment to those drug plans is based on adjustments to the national average of the plans' bids, not to an administratively calculated base payment amount as in Medicare Advantage.[16] Plan enrollees pay premiums composed of a "base amount" (a percentage of the nationwide average bid), plus or minus any difference between each plan's bid and the nationwide average. The bidding system was successfully implemented in two years—a major administrative accomplishment by the CMS, but also suggestive of the practicality of competitive pricing when the effort does not face crippling political or legal opposition.

As in other Medicare competitive pricing attempts, political pressures from the pharmaceutical industry played a substantial role in the Part D bidding design—notably, in restricting Part D provision to private plans and otherwise prohibiting any government role in the negotiation of prices. These two features have been the main objects of complaint from critics, although they were supported by a large body of independent opinion, not just the pharmaceutical industry.[17] These disputes are irrelevant for current purposes. The important issue here is that the system has been successful in setting the payments and premiums for Part D since 2006, with little complaint about the fact that it is competitive pricing. This begs the question of why it has been a political success when all the competitive pricing demonstrations have failed.

We don't have a definitive political analysis to offer, but two aspects of the Part D experience seem obviously important. First, the Part D bidding system was designed for a new benefit, rather than for an existing one. To appreciate why this matters, one need only do a simple thought experiment. Imagine that the Part D benefit already existed, with an administrative pricing system in place, creating a large, influential group—in this case, the pharmaceutical industry and benefit managers—with a vested interest in that system. The efficiencies of competitive pricing translate into lost revenue for those who benefit from administrative pricing.[18] The politics of that discussion would look a lot different from those surrounding competitive pricing for drugs in the MMA.

That leads to the second point, inferred above: the importance of limiting the benefit to private plans and restricting the government's role in negotiating drug prices. Whether or not one agrees with these provisions, they may have prevented the kind of political and legal opposition that has hindered past competitive pricing efforts by removing from the system what were, to industry, the most threatening options.

Unfortunately, what made Part D successful may well make it an inappropriate comparison for competitive pricing for MA plans and FFS—which are existing benefits with administrative pricing systems in place. Though few independent analysts take issue with the policy justifications for competitive bidding, the politics of changing an existing Medicare benefit are so difficult that few organizations appear to believe it is practical to propose it.

The Rule: Failures in Demonstrations for Existing Services

Apart from Part D, Medicare has a dismal record in attempts to introduce competitive pricing. No other Medicare benefit is now offered under competitive bidding, and all of the other efforts to establish it ultimately have failed under industry pressure, using beneficiary concerns as leverage.

As was shown in table 6-1, above, five competitive pricing demonstrations got to the point of bid evaluation: the two acute care demonstrations (CABG and ophthalmic); the second DME demonstration; and the first HMO demonstration (in Denver). All saved or promised to save substantial amounts of money. Three demonstrations got to the point of payment for services: the two acute care demonstrations and the second DME demonstration. None of these cases revealed beneficiary harms deriving from the bidding model. For example, the evaluation of the second DME demonstration concluded that beneficiary access and quality of services were essentially unchanged (U.S. Department of Health and Human Services 2004). It is important to emphasize that, if there had been any notable harms, they would have been documented, dramatized, and publicized by demonstration opponents, so the absence of evidence here is telling. The U.S. Government Accountability Office (2004) did note ways in which the CMS could improve the bidding model, but these improvements (such as the need to collect more information about the particular equipment being provided) were areas in which quality had more or less been taken for granted prior to the demonstration—that is, these improvements had nothing to do with competitive pricing as such, given that the same criticisms could be made of the traditional program. The fact that there is so little evidence of harm suggests that beneficiary harms are not the point.

Meanwhile, many of the demonstrations promised to improve provider quality, at least compared with Medicare's minimal, relatively unpoliced requirements for providers to qualify. For example, in the second DME demonstration, bidders had to qualify on certain special attributes related to quality. When the DME competitive bidding program was set to roll out nationwide, enhanced supplier standards were part of the bargain (U.S. Department of Health and Human Services, Centers for Medicare and Medicaid Services 2008). Some DME suppliers complained that they had been excluded for "paperwork problems," as if the issue were too much bureaucracy and complex regulations. The CMS investigated the complaints from a sample of one hundred companies and concluded that the disqualifications were justified because these companies had failed to meet quality standards for the bidding (Mathews 2008).

This episode suggests an important point about quality issues in competitive bidding. Quality monitoring, oversight, and incentives under conventional Medicare payment arrangements generally are weak, and often involve only initial qualification. The quality issues raised by the providers in competitive bidding had not received much consideration prior to the demonstration. Congress and the courts should be wary of newfound interest in quality, particularly on the part of health plans, suppliers, or providers, when competitive purchasing is introduced.

Competitive Pricing Works in Other Government-Financed Health-Care Programs

We know from Part D that competitive pricing is administratively practical. Meanwhile, as noted earlier, competitive pricing is commonplace in other government-financed health-care programs; the approach is used by most state Medicaid programs, the Veterans Administration (for instance, for basic oxygen and much DME), the Department of Defense (for the large and complex TRICARE solicitations), the Federal Employees Health Benefit Program (to select health plans for federal employees around the country), and the employee health benefit programs of many state governments. The problem is not that "government can't run these programs." While some government-run bidding programs are not administered very well (for some examples, see Whitford 2007), and while all such programs face administrative challenges (for example, see the analysis of TRICARE implementation issues in U.S. Government Accountability Office 2005), performance in general at every level of government has been sufficient to maintain widespread commitments to competitive bidding to set prices in publicly financed programs.

The political interests of health plans, providers, and others pose great difficulty in all large public health-care programs, and all public programs have to satisfy legal requirements that can limit discretion and be quite cumbersome at times. But these business interests seem to pose an insurmountable barrier to competitive bidding efforts only in Medicare, when the CMS attempts to convert from administrative prices. While Robert Reischauer is surely correct when he suggests that "there is really no political constituency for competition" in Medicare (Freudenheim 2003), sufficient constituency for price competition clearly exists in every other public health-care program of consequence. The question thus has to be, "Why not Medicare?"

Is Medicare Different?

We are not experts on Medicare politics, but it will be useful here to suggest the outlines of an answer to the question of why Medicare is different. Part of the answer is obvious: Medicare is different because of unique characteristics of the program. First, many health plans, suppliers, and providers have their entire market at stake. Medicare is the largest single payer for health services overall, and the Medicare market share is even more dominant in certain specialized areas (such as DME). As a result, the stakes are higher for these business interests, and they are ready to fight to keep from having to do in Medicare what they have to do routinely for other payers. As was recently noted with respect to the fight by suppliers to kill the DME competitive bidding program:

> Medicare spends billions of dollars each year on products and services that are available at far lower prices from retail pharmacies and online stores, according to an analysis of federal data by the *New York Times*. The government agency has paid above-market costs for dozens of items, a comparison of Medicare figures with retail catalogs finds . . .
>
> These widespread price discrepancies, including those for oxygen services, have been noted in dozens of regulatory reports.
>
> But when officials and politicians have tried to cut these costs, they have often encountered a powerful foe: the companies that sell these devices, who ask their elderly customers to serve, in effect, as unpaid lobbyists, calling and writing to their representatives in Congress, protesting at rallies, and even participating in political attacks against individual lawmakers who take on the issue.
>
> As the nation's elderly population grows, dozens of industries have tried to harness the political might of older Americans

for corporate goals. Physician groups, medical device manufacturers, insurance companies and other businesses have rallied aging voters to protest even minor legislative changes.

"These industries rely on a basic threat: If you mess with us, we can turn the seniors against you," said former Senator Alan K. Simpson, Republican of Wyoming, who tried cutting Medicare payments while he was in Congress. "Angering seniors is the quickest route to political suicide." (Duhigg 2007)

Second, Medicare beneficiaries are an especially sympathetic and politically important group. Medicare beneficiaries are old relative to the rest of the population, many of them are physically and mentally frail or financially vulnerable, and some are defenseless (or easy to depict as defenseless). Providers, suppliers, health plans, and others are quick to dramatize any conjectured potential for harm to beneficiaries. At the same time, the elderly are an important political bloc on their own. For purposes of political action by advocates and others, "the elderly" are not frail or defenseless.

The legal and political systems are sensitive to the claims elders make or that can be made on their behalf. For example, in the most recent clinical lab bidding attempt, a federal judge in San Diego was responsive to industry claims that competitive bidding would cause irreparable harm to Medicare patients.[19] The courts and the political establishment obviously have special deference for Medicare beneficiaries (for example, compared with the lesser sensitivity to Medicaid's relatively indigent, noninstitutional population), and so does the program. No one would disagree that it is thus hard to change anything in Medicare—such as the existing administrative pricing system for MA plans.

We should be careful, however, with explanations that assert that point and stop. Consider, for example, that the Department of Veterans Affairs has long used competitive bidding to acquire basic oxygen services for veterans (Coulam and Reardon 1990). This is a small market compared with Medicare, but the beneficiary group is politically powerful and elicits unique sympathies. Yet bidding is allowed to work in that context as a matter of course. Moreover, it is worth pointing out that the politics of Medicare payments seem to favor the status quo (whatever it is) more than a particular level of beneficence to all beneficiaries or areas of the country.

Health plans in high-payment areas seem able to block demonstrations that would change what they receive. But with the exception of the "floor" payment counties in the MA program, health plans and providers in low-payment areas are not necessarily able to acquire the same largesse for themselves.[20]

If Medicare were not in serious financial trouble, we would be inclined to agree that the status quo is likely to continue to preclude competitive bidding. But it is difficult to make this enormous concession to a vastly expensive status quo, just because Medicare issues are politically sensitive. Moreover, we should take some heart from the fact that, while the status quo is powerful, it is not as if Congress and the CMS never take on business interests in Medicare, even where the red herring of beneficiary interests can be raised. Consider just the three examples below.

The Tax Equity and Fiscal Responsibility Act of 1982 (TEFRA) and Prospective Payment System (PPS). The HCFA was able to implement prospective payment against the initial opposition of the hospital industry, and the history of the PPS is instructive for any consideration of competitive bidding. As described in detail by Mayes and Berenson (2006), the successful passage of the PPS by Congress began with, first, large year-to-year increases in hospital costs, well above inflation, and, second, policymakers' concerns about the financial stability of Medicare and Social Security. Declining payroll taxes in the early 1980s threatened to exhaust the trust funds of the two programs. To shore up Social Security, which faced the more immediate problem, funds were borrowed from the hospital trust fund. In response, Congress passed TEFRA, which imposed "the most significant restrictions on Medicare payments to hospitals in the program's history" (ibid., 38). The TEFRA limits were "strategically effective" for the passage of the PPS, as the limits included the prospect of hospital expenditure caps, which the hospital industry "loathed" (ibid.). This gave Congress political leverage when the PPS was proposed. Mayes and Berenson note,

> Financial necessity, particularly the specter of imminent bankruptcy, is the mother of all kinds of major programmatic invention . . . Extraordinary political and fiscal circumstances opened a rare window of opportunity for a major policy change.

To capitalize on this opportunity, however, once senior congressional leaders and the Reagan administration were in agreement, "attention turned to buying off any opposition from the hospital industry" (2006, 42–44).

As in competitive bidding, it was easy to argue not only that providers would be harmed, but that beneficiaries would be harmed as well (by "patient dumping," capacity losses that would reduce patient access, and so on). Although demonstrations showed large savings, generally without harmful effects (Coulam and Gaumer 1991), hospital opposition had to be overcome. In particular, while nonprofit hospitals and the American Hospital Association were somewhat inclined to work out a deal on the PPS to avoid TEFRA controls, the nation's teaching hospitals were strongly opposed. To secure their support, Congress made the terms of the PPS more generous to them. This sweetening undercut somewhat the fiscal purpose of the reform, but it was a key to its political success.

Thus, government could pit one subset of providers against another to achieve the desired policy. The PPS stands as a striking example of how Congress can act decisively when a fiscal crisis arises—but, even then, opponents have to be bought off!

The Balanced Budget Act of 1997 (BBA). As noted by Levit and colleagues,

> The Medicare provisions of the BBA were Congress's response to projected depletion of the [hospital insurance] trust fund and Medicare spending growth that had exceeded private insurers' spending growth in every year between 1992 and 1997, sometimes by wide margins. (Levit et al. 2000, 124)

Broad worries prevailed about rates of cost growth and evidence of overpayments to HMOs, DME, clinical laboratory services, home health services, hospital outpatient services, and others (Mayes and Berenson 2006). The BBA enacted a series of reductions in payments and created new authority to undertake competitive pricing demonstrations for HMOs and Part B services. The latter, which led to the second DME competitive bidding demonstrations, was passed by the same Congress that forced the cancellation of the Baltimore and Denver HMO demonstrations. The effect of the HMO payment cuts was to squeeze payments in high-payment areas toward the norm, and to raise them in low-payment (largely rural) areas. Perhaps something about across-the-board cuts makes them politically easier than local demonstrations (see chapter 8). More interesting for our purposes, the BBA suggested that it is possible to subordinate Medicare to fiscal policy. Indeed, "Medicare [was] the ultimate budgetary 'slush fund'. . . . The BBA represented the height of Medicare politics' subordination to fiscal partisan politics" (Mayes and Berenson, 2006, 104, 105). When fiscal problems are imminent, and the politics tractable, Congress can be prompted to act against business interests, at least temporarily, to bring high payments under control.

The Second DME Demonstration. This is the closest Medicare has come to successful implementation of competitive bidding for an *existing* service. In launching the demonstration, one key factor was the chance support of key politicians. (The opposition of politicians representing the demonstration sites had crippled other demonstrations.) Thus, as described by Dowd and others (2000), Senator Bob Graham (D-Florida), the author of the BBA amendment that mandated competitive bidding demonstrations for DME and other Part B services, remained a steadfast supporter of the approach. In a press release after Polk County, Florida, was chosen as the first site for the DME demonstration, Senator Graham "hailed the establishment of the Polk County pilot project" and was quoted as saying,

> In the past, Medicare was forced to purchase medical supplies and services in a manner better suited to the communist systems of old—with pre-set prices, complicated rules, without competition. I am very proud that Polk County will be leading Medicare into a new era where market forces keep prices low and help to preserve this crucial health care program for our children and grandchildren. (Graham 1998, 1)

Meanwhile, Florida governor Lawton Chiles strongly supported the demonstration. In a letter to the HCFA administrator, he expressed his pleasure that the HCFA had

> selected Florida as a test site for a project to help protect the Medicare program. I extend my full cooperation and support to

[the HCFA administrator] and HCFA for this important initiative. (Chiles 1998, 1)

These reactions stand in marked contrast to the opposition, often immediate and *extraordinarily* vehement, from legislators of both parties representing areas where unsuccessful competitive pricing demonstrations were attempted for Medicare HMOs—for example, Senators Kyl of Arizona, Nighthorse-Campbell of Colorado, Ashcroft of Missouri, and Mikulski of Maryland.

These three examples are instructive. First, they suggest that Medicare and general government finances can reach a point that compels Congress to act. Second, credible threats of congressional action can bring industry groups to the table, as when the TEFRA legislation made hospitals more willing to consider the PPS. Third, even when there is a fiscal crisis, it is essential to divide industry groups by buying them off (at least, a sufficient bloc of them) to reduce their opposition to difficult payment reforms. Fourth, the vigorous support of key political leaders is essential. That support may come by chance, or there may be ways to encourage it.

Challenges to Future Competitive Pricing Efforts

All of these examples point to the challenges to the future success of competitive pricing efforts, as we discuss below.

Administrative Complexity. Competitive pricing is practical, and the CMS has demonstrated that it is perfectly capable of administering a competitive pricing system for a complex drug benefit and for MA plans. But administration is not easy. As noted by Christianson over twenty years ago (1987, 85), "It is recognized in the literature that 'contracting entails substantial administrative costs.'" Or, as noted by Coulam,

To all who participate in them, [competitive bidding] processes are extremely labor intensive, demanding substantial involvement of management at every level and opening an agency to threats (legal, political, and other) from virtually every party to the transactions involved. (Coulam, 1995, 1)

In complex processes, the CMS, like all other administrators, occasionally makes mistakes. Opponents have used such mistakes in competitive bidding efforts as pretexts to halt the demonstrations in court. For example, in the recent San Diego case on clinical laboratory bidding, a judge concluded that the CMS had failed to follow notice and comment procedures required by the 1946 Administrative Procedures Act, a failure that added credibility to the industry's claim that harms had not been fully anticipated. A Denver judge reached similar conclusions in a challenge brought to stop the first HMO demonstration. As summarized by the GAO, health plans in Denver argued that

> the addition of a requirement that plans must participate in a competitive bidding demonstration as a condition of receiving or renewing a Medicare contract amounts to a change in the current Medicare regulations governing HMO participation that is unlawful because it is being made outside the normal rule-making process . . . the existing demonstration authority does not relieve HCFA of its obligation to meet the requirements of the rule-making process if the agency wishes to condition the renewal or issuance of Medicare HMO contracts on participation in the demonstration. (U.S. General Accounting Office 1997, 9)

The judge agreed with the plans, granting a temporary restraining order,[21] after which the parties entered into a joint stipulation for dismissal, wherein the U.S. Department of Health and Human Services agreed to terminate the demonstration project immediately (Barnes 2005).

A different kind of procedural glitch based on a simple administrative mistake, rather than on legal complexities, occurred in the second HMO bidding demonstration. At a key juncture, the CMS missed the deadline for publishing notice of a meeting of the Kansas City advisory committee in the *Federal Register*. This meant the next meeting could not take place until a month later, thus giving opponents of the demonstration in both the Kansas City and Phoenix sites more time to organize (Dowd et al. 2000).

Three things should be noted about these procedural problems. First, procedural protections serve important functions in an orderly government, but they are being used here as a pretext to obstruct more efficient purchasing of government-financed services. Second, industry claims of disruption do not always dupe judges. In the second DME demonstration rollout, judges twice refused to grant injunctions that the DME industry requested. The industry then went to Congress, which acted on the complaints. Third, inadequate administrative resources, including legal support, make administrative mistakes more likely.

Consideration may be necessary of the statutory framework for competitive bidding and the claims that can be entertained to obstruct it. Given the administrative demands of competitive bidding, the CMS may need to devote more legal resources to it.

Willingness of Health Plans, Suppliers, and Others to Accept Flat Cuts to Avoid Competitive Pricing. In at least three of the demonstrations (the first DME demonstration, the first HMO demonstration, and the second clinical lab demonstration), supplier and health plan representatives stated a preference for flat cuts in reimbursement to a competitive bidding regime. This industry response is a challenge to the success of competitive bidding for two reasons. First, it illustrates the lengths to which the industry is willing to go to avoid competitive bidding. Second, it is an option that politicians might accept, as a compromise that saves some money and avoids antagonizing industry.

In Denver, in meetings before bids in the first HMO demonstration were to be submitted, an industry representative offered to the CMS: "What do you want? Ten percent? Fifteen percent? Why don't you just tell us how much you want to cut the price?"[22] In the first DME demonstration, the industry avoided competitive bidding by agreeing to a fee schedule that incorporated a cut in payments for oxygen services (Coulam et al. 1990). In 2008, in the phased national program of DME competitive bidding, industry acceded to a 10 percent cut in fees to get the delay in competitive bidding:

> The industry . . . is looking to Congress to scrap the competitive bidding program being put in place by [the CMS], which the agency projects will reduce Medicare's DME spending by 26 percent. The $6 billion, five-year cost of getting rid of that is prohibitive, [Representative Stark, chair of the Subcommittee on Health of the Ways and Means Committee] suggested.

The industry has loudly complained about the way CMS selected the winning bidders in the first 10 metropolitan areas and charged that competitive bidding would drive suppliers out of the market and reduce access for beneficiaries.

Stark indicated he'd heard those concerns and suggested an alternative: keeping the program's new quality standards and using the bid prices to set lower, national fee rates but doing away with the bidding itself. That could turn out to be the industry's worst nightmare. (Young 2008)

The irony of using bid prices to reduce the fee schedules to pay for the elimination of the competitive bidding that revealed the lower prices in the first place apparently was lost. *This is a critical issue:* The only way for the CMS and Congress to know what the appropriately lower prices would be is to use competitive bidding to reveal the underlying costs of efficient, qualified producers.

Industry agreed to large cuts in these cases to avoid having to compete on price. Suppliers and health plans evidently prefer benefit/service competition within Medicare's generous (or even reduced) prices to price competition within a fixed benefit. A sure sign that suppliers and health plans are overpaid—and that competitive bidding works to reduce prices—is the alacrity with which these business interests agree to large, across-the-board cuts to avoid the constant competitive pressure on prices from a bidding system.

Fears That Beneficiaries Will Be Harmed by Competitive Pricing. Reasonably disinterested critics may have a number of reasons to fear competitive pricing. The first is that competitive prices will lead to lower quality. In some ways, the political system is as comfortable as providers are with fixed, often generous prices. There is a widespread belief that generous prices encourage high quality, and that low-price health plans, suppliers, and providers offer low quality, perhaps in ways that cannot be observed.

In fact, there is no evidence that higher prices are consistently associated with higher quality, and some evidence that excess payments instead encourage fraud and abuse (Coulam et al. 1997). Those who fear that the quality of care will suffer as a result of competitive pricing also overrate the protections that exist under traditional administrative pricing arrangements.

The Medicare program is more or less passive in the face of unfavorable changes in the competitiveness of particular markets. Neither the CMS nor any other entity (such as the Joint Commission on the Accreditation of Healthcare Organizations) ensures that providers use excess payments to provide higher quality.

The second fear is that aggressive providers will low-ball their bids to drive the competition out of business and then use their increased market power to raise prices and reduce quality. While so-called predatory pricing is possible, we think it would be extremely rare among private Medicare health plans. In predatory pricing, a firm sells its product at a price below short-run marginal cost to drive its rivals out of business (Areeda and Turner 1975). For this tactic to be successful, the firm must have a high probability of recouping its losses. As Klevorick (1993) wrote, "The essence of predatory pricing is the sacrifice of short-term gains for longer-run gains." Private Medicare plans are unlikely to recoup their losses in the long run, first, because new firms could enter the market at a fairly small scale (see chapter 3) and keep prices low, and, second, as noted earlier, Medicare could use competitive arrangements to establish monitoring and reporting to detect the anticipated quality reductions.

In fact, rather than harming beneficiaries, competitive bidding arrangements provide a natural administrative platform for maintaining and enhancing competition and quality. For example, especially given politically potent worries about quality of care in competitive bidding, the establishment of additional qualification requirements for bidders (such as enhanced accreditation as a condition of bidding) and additional data requirements (such as enhanced monitoring of quality and access) may be desirable. The nationwide competitive bidding program for durable medical equipment included such enhancements (U.S. Government Accountability Office 2008). Any enhancements designed to improve quality in MA plans should be applied to FFS Medicare as well.

The primary interests being served by the obstruction of competitive bidding in Medicare are health plans' interests in maintaining excess payments. Medicare costs are health plan revenues, and plans do not want to lose them. Through bidder qualification and closer oversight, competitive pricing would bring scrutiny to areas of the Medicare benefit that currently get only cursory review. The industry would like to avoid that stricter oversight.[23]

Congress and the courts generally have been responsive to industry complaints. To far too great an extent, Medicare has become a provider/supplier/health plan welfare program (Cooper and Vladek 2000). Legitimate needs of providers and others to engage in orderly business with Medicare are one thing; entitlement to inflated prices is another matter. If there is to be any Medicare reform, the program must be able to pay no more than reasonable market prices for the services it covers.

Finally, we need to remember that large private employers have been running competitive pricing systems with multiple health plan offerings for decades. These systems have been relatively stable and have produced lower costs than alternatives, such as single-plan systems (Vistnes, Cooper, and Vistnes 2001).

What Is to Be Done?

We have no magic solution to the power of business interests, Congress, and the courts to maintain administrative pricing for existing Medicare services. But, as noted throughout this book, the need to control Medicare costs is increasingly urgent, making old arrangements more difficult to accept. If Medicare costs are to be controlled, the CMS needs legal and political space to implement competitive pricing. But we do not mean to end this argument by saying something as banal as "Medicare politics have to change," though clearly they do. We can see a number of smaller, practical steps that the CMS, Congress, and others can take to ease the political problem, though we are well aware that many of these, individually, have been unsuccessful.

Recognize that competitive pricing is one part of fixing Medicare's increasingly urgent fiscal problems. It seems obvious that political and legal cover for competitive pricing and the discretion it requires will come only when fiscal exigencies are deeply felt, and Congress connects those problems in part to the prices Medicare pays (as occurred in a smaller way in the passage of the Balanced Budget Act). Both political design (for example, the passage of TEFRA as a disliked alternative) and courage or luck (for example, the advocacy of Senator Graham) may be important.

Consider ways to divide health plan opposition or buy it off. Concessions were made to divide and reduce the opposition to the PPS. So it might be done here. For example, bidding rules can be manipulated to reduce political opposition—for instance, by choosing the average bid of a qualified health plan rather than the lowest bid, to reduce fears that low-priced health plans will drive high-quality plans out of business. This strategy can be very costly, however.[24]

Be aware that some bidding models might face fewer legal and political problems than others. We can't prove the point, but our sense is that Congress and the courts particularly dislike bidding models that exclude bidders directly through the bidding process itself, rather than through the consequences of the bidding (that is, through providers' inability to compete successfully). Thus, models that exclude losing bidders face particularly difficult political problems, as with DME, and legal problems in federal courts, as with clinical laboratory services. Of course, these models exclude losers for a reason (Karon et al. 2002).[25] But others do not, including the HMO model we propose, and that is an advantage. At the same time, some possible aspects of bidding may pose particularly serious threats to business interests, as in the case of the bidding models that used government buying power to set Part D drug prices. Compromise on those terms may reduce opposition.

Cultivate political leaders to support competitive bidding as a policy. Political leaders can oppose health plans effectively if they are committed to competitive bidding. In the DME case, political support came about by chance. But the CMS and supporters of competitive bidding in Congress should consider how to enhance such support. To some degree, this is a tautological solution—solve the political problem by getting political leaders not to oppose it. We are, however, suggesting something more active than wishful thinking. If competitive bidding is to be successful, we will need more Senator Grahams who embrace it for their own states, and that requires a strategy to build support.

Compensate losers, at least through a transition period. Competitive pricing means that someone has to lose, as highlighted in our estimates of loss or disruption in chapter 4. That loss provokes at least some of the political

opposition against competitive bidding. For example, the earlier HMO bidding demonstrations required budget neutrality at the site level, which
meant that the HCFA could not make the demonstration more worthwhile
for the areas selected to be guinea pigs—a point emphasized by Nichols
and Reischauer (2000). Some form of mitigating the losses might ease the
opposition. The benefits of that investment have to be balanced against the
costs. At some point, the policy is so undermined that the effort is not
worthwhile—for example, note the large reduction in savings that results
from using an average-bid competitive pricing model, versus a lowest-bid
model (see chapter 4). Unless it is the only way to get competitive pricing,
we find that cost too great for the benefits such a concession might bring.
In any event, calculations along these lines are inevitable when competitive
bidding is introduced.

*Tell beneficiaries now about the changes coming, and give them a long period to
adjust.* If beneficiary arrangements and expectations cannot be disrupted
without large political consequences, it is better to minimize the disruption by slowly bringing about major change rather than avoiding major
change altogether. This subject deserves special attention, which we give it
in chapter 8.

*Strengthen the administrative and legal resources available to the CMS in com-
petitive bidding struggles.* If administrative mistakes have been part of the
problem, one obvious recommendation is that the CMS be given more
administrative support to run these bidding programs. Moreover, it is not
clear to us that the agency has been well or aggressively defended against
lawsuits designed to obstruct competitive bidding programs. The government perhaps should have more specialized attorneys to defend these suits.

*Revise the legal framework to give the CMS more flexibility to run competitive
bidding programs.* The CMS needs more procedural flexibility to run a substantial competitive bidding program than current law allows. While procedural and substantive safeguards are necessary, it would be useful to
narrow the grounds for health plans and others to impede competitive bidding programs. In particular, for example, the potential beneficiary harms
that provide sufficient grounds to justify delay should be clearly defined, so

that something more than spectral worries is required to block competitive pricing efforts.

As competition raises particular fears about quality, bidding efforts should promise increases in quality to counter them. A number of reasonable fears have been raised about competitive pricing. The CMS could address them more directly by using more aggressive processes of quality measurement and monitoring. If a decline in quality in unobserved dimensions as a result of competitive bidding is a concern, then the CMS should make efforts to increase what is being observed. For example, the GAO noted that DME suppliers in competitive bidding and in the traditional, fee-schedule system need only provide Healthcare Common Procedure Coding System (HCPCS) codes to describe the items of equipment they provide, and that a single HCPCS code can cover widely differing items (U.S. Government Accountability Office 2004).[26] Any effort to understand the effects of competitive bidding on changes in the quality of equipment would require a more refined coding system. The CMS could not revamp the intricate HCPCS coding system when it expanded competitive bidding nationwide, but it did make special efforts to enhance quality. As noted by the GAO,

> For the competitive bidding program, CMS required suppliers to obtain accreditation based on quality standards and provide financial documents to participate . . . This added scrutiny gives CMS the chance to screen out suppliers that may not be stable, legitimate businesses, which could contribute to lower rates of improper payment. (U.S. Government Accountability Office 2008, i)

To be sure, this process of screening out suppliers has a downside, as was also apparent in the DME bidding program: Suppliers who are screened out cry foul, and make politically compelling arguments that beneficiaries are going to lose access (see, for example, Wayne 2008).

Three important themes underlie all of the suggestions we have discussed here: the need to take opposition seriously and act to reduce it; a skepticism of the comfort we should have with the quality of services or care the FFS system provides and a sense of the possibilities for improvements that are created when the program establishes orderly bidding arrangments with more active quality monitoring; and, finally, the need to consider competitive bidding more seriously at a time when the Medicare program faces dire financial threats.

7

No Need for a Demonstration—
A Gradual Transition to Reform
Should Start Now

In this chapter, we argue that there is no need to demonstrate competitive pricing because we know enough already to conclude that it will work. Demonstrations that affect some Medicare beneficiaries also are likely to be more controversial than national reform that affects all beneficiaries equally. Instead of a demonstration, we recommend a gradual transition to competitive pricing that recognizes legitimate beneficiary interests.

Given our analysis of the four options for Medicare payment policy, and given our view of what is required to serve the purposes of the Medicare program, we have concluded that competitive pricing is the most desirable option. A demonstration of this concept would, therefore, seem logical; and, in fact, one is scheduled to begin in 2010. In this chapter, however, we argue that the demonstration is not necessary, and that we should proceed directly to implementing competitive pricing on a national scale. We don't need a demonstration of competitive pricing because, first, we already know almost everything that could be learned from one, and, second, demonstrations that affect only a subset of Medicare beneficiaries appear to be more controversial than program-wide changes that affect all beneficiaries. We consider these issues in turn.

What We Know Already about Competitive Pricing Makes a Demonstration Unnecessary

In addition to knowledge gained through the experience of large employers with competitive pricing systems, consider what we know already about competitive pricing in Medicare.

We know that some managed-care plans will submit bids lower than comparable FFS costs. As noted earlier, in the previous attempt to demonstrate competitive pricing for HMOs, the bids from four of the eight M+C plans in Denver were 24–38 percent below the published BBA payment rates for 1998 (Dowd 2001). We would expect similar results if competitive bidding were hosted by a market such as Denver, with an above-average M+C payment rate and a competitive HMO market.

We know that competitive pricing is administratively feasible. In Denver, Medicare speedily prepared and issued instructions for competitive bidding, and health plans responded with little difficulty (Dowd, Coulam, and Feldman 2000). Possibly more to the point, Medicare implemented competitive pricing for prescription drug benefits *nationally* in 2006 with great success. We know that it can be done for health plans.

Competitive bidding also has shown impressive demonstration results for one Medicare benefit—durable medical equipment (DME)—as discussed in chapter 6. Though DME is a small part of the Medicare benefit, bidding for it was a major challenge, resolved successfully and without notable effects on access or quality.

We know a great deal about the quality of care in managed-care plans. Dowd and Feldman concluded, "More is known about the quality of care in FFS Medicare versus M+C plans than in any other health insurance sector" (2002, 212). There is no systematic empirical support for the concern that managed-care plans skimp on quality for Medicare beneficiaries or that care is superior in FFS Medicare. We share MedPAC's concerns, however, that newer plans (for which market entry became economical at the current high payment rates for MA plans) have lower clinical quality of care than older plans,[1] and that private fee-for-service plans are exempt from reporting quality measures. Like MedPAC, we also are concerned that FFS Medicare is exempt from reporting quality measures (U.S. Medicare Payment Advisory Commission 2008a, 238). Competitive pricing might improve quality of care if it "weeds out" inefficient plans or plan types that cannot deliver good quality for the lowest cost. Finally, as noted in chapter 6, we agree with the GAO that the CMS should use the occasion of competitive pricing to undertake special quality-monitoring efforts (U.S. Government Accountability Office 2004), if only to provide reassurance against fears raised by opponents.

We know who will be disrupted by competitive pricing and approximately how much. Disruption will occur in local markets where the FFS bid is substantially lower (this is also true of MedPAC's and the Obama administration's proposals that remove payment "floors") or higher than the lowest bid from a qualified private plan. Valuable information about the first type of disruption was produced by the BBA during the period 1998–2004, in which payments to private Medicare health plans were limited in many markets, leading to disruptive reductions in MA benefits, increased out-of-pocket premiums, and plan exits from the market. From this experience, we know that HMOs will leave Medicare when payments are cut, but payment isn't the plans' only consideration. During the BBA period, plans' decisions to stay or drop counties also varied by year and by their national-firm affiliations (Halpern 2005). On average, a $100 decrease in payment (about 20 percent of the mean) increased the probability of dropping a county in 1999–2000 by three percentage points.

Schoenman and colleagues (2005) assessed the experiences of Medicare beneficiaries who were involuntarily disenrolled when their HMOs exited from six Medicare markets between 1998 and 1999. Many dealt with the transition without disruption, but minorities and those with lower income and education were more likely to know less about their health insurance options. Some beneficiaries said they were no longer able to see their physicians after disenrollment, and 4 percent reported not seeking desired or needed care after losing their HMOs. In another study, Parente and others (2005) compared health-care use and cost among Medicare beneficiaries who were involuntarily disenrolled from their HMOs between 1998 and 1999 and returned to FFS with those who voluntarily left their HMOs.

Involuntarily disenrolled beneficiaries had higher out-of-pocket expenditures, more emergency room use, and a higher probability of dying. Finally, when HMOs leave, the odds of beneficiaries being "very concerned" about getting care they need are directly related to having limited or no HMO managed-care penetration in their counties (Booske et al. 2002).

Natural experiments like the BBA don't provide guidance on what would happen if the out-of-pocket premium for FFS Medicare were to increase by a large amount, as is likely in at least some market areas under competitive pricing. However, several observational studies (Buchmueller 2000; Atherly, Dowd, and Feldman 2004; Pizer, Frakt, and Feldman 2007) have estimated the probability that beneficiaries will stay in FFS or switch to private plans when the FFS premium increases. The findings from these studies indicate that a large premium increase would be necessary before a significant amount of switching occurred.[2] This evidence suggests that higher FFS premiums will result in financial disruption, as most beneficiaries who are affected will opt to pay the higher premiums and have less disposable income to spend on other goods and services. Lower-income beneficiaries probably will be the most likely to leave FFS Medicare, but Thorpe and Atherly's data (2002) suggest that many of them already have left.

In summary, some beneficiaries would be disrupted by competitive pricing, and some private plans would exit from Medicare. While the overall level of disruption should be within manageable limits, the impact of private plan exits would be concentrated among vulnerable groups, and the disruption from higher FFS premiums would be felt most strongly by low-income beneficiaries who remained in FFS Medicare. But this is true of all the options to current Medicare payment policy. There will be no acceptable alternative to the current payment policy if no more than *minimal* beneficiary disruption is allowed. In any event, the key question here is whether, in the current fiscal climate, a discussion about how to pay MA plans should be stalemated by the prospect of some disruption to some groups that may require protection. We argue that it takes very little imagination to figure out reasonable, more efficient ways to hold such groups harmless, and that in almost every case it will be less expensive to do that than to subsidize more generous coverage for everyone so that some may be spared.

The Controversy of a Demonstration

Paradoxically, it may be politically easier to implement competitive pricing as a national reform with no demonstration. Demonstrations single out groups of beneficiaries and treat them differently from their peers. When the changes being tested have a significant effect on all the major stakeholders in a particular site, demonstrations may be impossible. It is easy to mobilize "not in my backyard" sentiments to block a demonstration before it can be started when some areas appear unfairly singled out. Unsurprisingly, congressional delegations are responsive to those appeals. Both Republicans and Democrats rose up to block the previous competitive pricing demonstration for HMOs in all four cities.[3] Efforts to kill the 2010 CCA demonstration are underway.[4]

The Case for Gradualism

In the preceding chapters, we explained why competitive pricing is desirable, but we also concluded there is no easy solution to the problem of Medicare payment policy, especially if policymakers insist that reforms only minimally disrupt beneficiaries. Here we argue that the benefit of moving toward a sustainable payment system in the long run might withstand complaints about disruption if, but likely *only* if, we tell beneficiaries, health plans, and others now what that system will be; if we insist on maintaining that goal in the face of inevitable complaints (delay can't be allowed simply to provide time for opponents to build opposition to the program); and if we move toward it gradually, allowing stakeholders to adjust their expectations and arrangements without abrupt changes.

The gradual movement toward a new system could be accomplished in one of at least two ways. First, Congress could pick a future year for full implementation and then, over the transition period, blend new and old methods in a gradual shift to the new. There are many technical issues to consider, but the essential point is that full application of the new method would not occur *anywhere* until a definite year in the future. Second, the new method could be implemented more or less immediately, but Medicare could provide buffers for those areas where it causes substantial change (for instance, more than 5 percent). Under this approach, in many areas the adjustment could be rather quick, but in areas where FFS or private plans have a substantial cost advantage (areas prone to the greatest disruption), the phase-in could be longer. This form of transition has some precedents,[5] but the more common version of a gradual transition is the first one: to pick a year of full implementation and gradually move toward it everywhere.

We know of at least two major Medicare payment reforms—the physician fee schedule for Part B and risk-adjusted payments to Medicare HMOs—that ultimately were successful and that used the "target date" form of gradualism. While neither example is an exact analogy or a guide to the likely success of phasing in competitive pricing for Medicare health plans, the two reforms share some interesting similarities. Both were responses to widely held perceptions that the existing methods for paying doctors and health plans weren't working. Prior to 1992, the perceived cost of providing physician services was too high and was spiraling upward rapidly (Antos 1991). In response, Congress replaced the old method of paying physicians (based on comparing their submitted charges to screens for what would be reasonable) with a new fee schedule. The original impetus for risk-adjusted HMO payments was that the payment cells based on enrollees' demographic characteristics were too crude, and that HMOs were "cherry-picking" the least expensive enrollees within each payment cell (Brown et al. 1993). The impetus for later modifications to the risk adjustment system, however, was that the earlier versions were based on data collected in the hospital, and MA plans were trying hard to reduce unnecessary hospitalizations.

Both reforms featured long phase-in periods because the affected stakeholders blocked speedier implementation. Established by the Omnibus Budget Reconciliation Act of 1989, the Part B fee schedule was phased in over a four-year period starting on January 1, 1992, because of opposition from procedure-oriented specialists whose fees would be reduced. Risk-adjusted payments for HMOs began in 2000, but full implementation was delayed until 2007 because of "clashes with the managed care industry over payment policy, concerns over perverse incentives, and problems of data burden" (Weissman, Wachterman, and Blumenthal 2005, 475). Once the system was implemented, it was a major improvement over the old method of risk adjustment. The notable feature of these reforms is that both eventually were implemented, opposition notwithstanding.

There is also at least one example of a Medicare reform that directly affected beneficiaries and was implemented over a relatively brief phase-in period: means-testing of Part B premiums as required by the Medicare Modernization Act (P.L. 108-173). This reform seems to be proceeding smoothly, although it is too early to judge its ultimate success. In our opinion, however, it is not a good model for implementing competitive pricing for Medicare health plans. Unlike means-tested Part B premiums, which affect only a small fraction of upper-income beneficiaries, competitive pricing will affect many beneficiaries, including those with low incomes. Hence the importance of a gradual phase-in of competitive pricing: An abrupt phase-in of competitive bidding would be unlikely to allow enough time for beneficiaries to make alternative arrangements, such as saving enough money to pay the extra premiums for FFS in some areas, or finding new doctors if their HMOs leave the program in response to dramatic payment cuts.

Even a gradual phase-in of competitive pricing might not be able to prevent HMOs from leaving the Medicare program immediately to avoid future payment reductions. Medicare might wish to cushion the disruption from HMO exits by providing assistance to enrollees who need to change doctors. For example, Medicare could publicize which physicians were accepting new FFS patients. This information could be tailored to the specific needs of the beneficiary groups most likely to be disrupted by competitive pricing. Given enough time, beneficiaries would adjust to the changes implied by competitive pricing, including the decision that the added costs of their preferred alternative are not worth paying.

An example of an unsuccessful attempt to phase in a new payment system for Medicare health plans were the BBA payment reforms of 1997. The BBA methods were phased in by blending so-called national and local payment amounts with a year-by-year increase in the proportion of the national amount. The effect was a compression in rates. The political pushback from beneficiaries and plans was felt first in certain moderating amendments in 1999 and 2000, followed by a more radical change in 2003, as Congress pushed for a larger role for private plans in the MMA. Needless to say, while the BBA is not exactly analogous to the competitive pricing reform we propose here—among other things, FFS beneficiaries were not affected directly—it stands as a caution that gradualism is not a cure-all, especially if political sentiments shift against reform. As we consider the possibility of competitive pricing and political push-back, perhaps the most important difference from the BBA experience is the increased fiscal stress on the Medicare program, which makes the current case for competitive pricing more compelling.

Conclusion

Our goal in this book was to design a payment system for Medicare health plans. But we also offered our vision for reform of the *entire* Medicare program. In our view, Medicare should have a defined-benefit package (set by the people's elected representatives) that is offered to all beneficiaries by at least one health plan in every market area for no more than the Part B premium. Medicare currently has a defined-benefit package that is offered to all beneficiaries for no more than the Part B premium, but it is offered by a particular health plan—FFS Medicare. The amounts paid for this plan, with various additions and subtractions, depending on the political temperament of the times, have determined how much private plans in the Medicare program will be paid. We do not think this is a rational, stable, fiscally responsible, or fair payment system.

Our vision of Medicare includes both private Medicare plans and the public plan. Some would dispute this vision, arguing that the public plan or private plans should have the exclusive franchise for Medicare. We disagree because the public plan and private plans both have advantages and disadvantages. We explained this position in chapter 1.

Different Congresses and administrations have, however, tilted the playing field in favor of one plan type or another with what seem to be predictable reversals. In the BBA era, private plans suffered reduced payment rates, and many left the Medicare program. In the post-MMA era, the pendulum has swung decisively in the other direction, and private plans are favored over the public plan. These changes in favoritism consume resources needlessly and are disruptive to beneficiaries. They also substitute the political decisions for those of health plans and beneficiaries throughout the rest of the country. It is time to design a payment system that, first, lets plans tell the government how much they want to be paid, not the other way around; and, second, subjects them to a predictable set of consequences if they submit low or high bids.

A competitive pricing system would use plans' bids to determine the government payment rate for all Medicare plans, including FFS Medicare. Our preferred form of competitive pricing would rely on the low bid from any plan to set the payment rate, subject to having enough capacity in a low-bidding plan of adequate quality to handle its expected enrollment. Other versions of competitive pricing, however, relying on some function of the bids, would be available as well. The reward for low bidders would be increased enrollment; the penalty for high bidders would be charging an out-of-pocket premium, which would drive beneficiaries away for a good reason—they are more costly than their competitors!

We explored the technical issues in setting up a competitive pricing system for Medicare, and we argued that a demonstration of competitive pricing is not necessary. Large public and private employers that offer multiple health plans have been using competitive pricing for years, with favorable results.

Notwithstanding our conviction that competitive pricing is essential to Medicare reform, we are well aware that we are arguing against a frustrating history of competitive pricing in Medicare. The new Part D benefit is an exception that proves the rule: There have been no successful attempts to introduce competitive pricing as a replacement for administrative prices *that have already created politically powerful winners from the overpayments inevitable in those systems.* We have no magic solution to this opposition. Based on previous competitive pricing efforts and on Medicare initiatives in other areas, however, we can mention a few modest approaches that would help to reduce that opposition, including

- recognizing that competitive pricing is one part of fixing Medicare's increasingly urgent fiscal problems;

- devising ways to divide the health plan opposition or buy it off;

- seeking bidding models whose features tend to provoke somewhat less opposition; and

- preparing beneficiaries and buffering them from any substantial or abrupt effects.

Finally, competitive pricing can be used in ways that will enhance the quality of care and reduce fears that competition will hurt beneficiaries. The political system that fears the quality effects of competitive pricing is, in fact, quite complacent about the quality provided by an only modestly monitored FFS program. By contrast, the contractual platform that competitive pricing creates can ensure careful monitoring and the maintenance of quality.

In all of this, we need to appreciate that most criticisms of competitive pricing are products of self-interest camouflaged in attractively elevated principles, such as protecting beneficiaries, promoting access, and assisting the indigent. Medicare can serve these other objectives at lower cost in other ways than through the payment system. It is of critical importance now that the government get its contributions right, and competitive pricing is the only system that can do that.

Our competitive pricing proposal could save about 8 percent of Medicare costs, *more than any other payment reform now under consideration for health plans.* Saving even 8 percent will not solve Medicare's financial problems. But if we are to solve those problems, we will at least need to get the payments right.

Everyone agrees that Medicare must do something to control costs, and our proposal is a step in that direction. Moreover, of all the payment-reform proposals, it is the only one that will remove the subsidies that distort the government's decisions regarding the Medicare entitlement benefit package, end political bickering over administratively determined Medicare Advantage payments, and stabilize payment policy for Medicare health plans. These are powerful advantages, at a time when the program badly needs them.

Notes

Introduction

1. Medicare also covers younger adults with permanent disabilities, but we do not discuss that part of the program—comprising approximately 16 percent of all enrollees—in this book, as the payment and provider arrangements for that group are sufficiently different to require separate treatment.

2. For a more complete program description, see Kaiser Family Foundation (2009), from which the following brief overview is drawn.

3. The Medicare tax is part of the Federal Insurance Contributions Act (FICA) tax. The tax rates currently are 1.45 percent each for employers and employees.

4. See U.S. Medicare Payment Advisory Commission 2009, chapter 3, for a discussion of enhanced benefits offered by MA plans. Part C premiums are set annually through a process we will describe later.

5. See Williams (2005) for a concise discussion of these goals.

6. Of course, these claims for Medicare Advantage are contested. For example, see Families USA 2007b.

7. It may not be obvious how FFS Medicare can "bid" within a competitive pricing system. We will have more to say on this later. The main ideas to have in mind at this stage are that, first, standardized average FFS costs in a geographic area would be calculated and compared with MA bids; second, the benchmark price would be set (for instance, based on the lowest bid, the average bid, or the median); and third, all bids (including FFS) would be compared to the benchmark. FFS would be treated like any other plan. Thus, if the FFS bid were greater than the benchmark, beneficiaries would have to pay an additional premium if they wished to enroll in FFS. If the FFS bid were less than the benchmark, then beneficiaries would get some extra benefits—for example, in the form of a reduction in their Part B premium.

8. As reported by Freudenheim (2003), "Similar plans [to the CCA] . . . have failed to find support among patients, doctors and hospitals, or even some insurers. Even people who favor the idea say the potential for trouble this time is formidable. 'There is really no political constituency for competition,' said Robert D. Reischauer, a health policy expert and a former director of the Congressional Budget Office."

9. The CCA demonstration is scheduled to begin in at least six metropolitan areas on January 1, 2010. FFS Medicare will be required to compete with MA plans, with a single weighted-average bid being calculated from the FFS bid and MA plans' bids.

Chapter 1: The Purposes of Medicare

1. Our views on this topic have been published previously in Dowd et al. (2005–6) and Berenson and Dowd (2008).

2. Universal availability of private plans was achieved in 2006 through a combination of regional and local PPOs, HMOs, and private fee-for-service (PFFS) plans. Starting in 2007, PFFS plans have been universally available. Regional PPOs were established by the 2003 MMA legislation. Their service areas are defined by the CMS and cover both rural and urban areas, and each must serve an entire region. Regional PPOs are offered a financial incentive to enter the market and a further subsidy if they enroll a disproportionate number of beneficiaries from rural counties (Pizer, Frakt, and Feldman 2007). They are subject to some additional requirements: They must offer a combined Part A and Part B deductible (if applicable) and a cap on out-of-pocket spending. However, "they have greater flexibility in meeting provider access standards and in establishing cost sharing requirements for in-network and out-of-network providers" (National Health Policy Forum 2005, 2).

3. To be sure, there are minor geographic variations in the entitlement. For example, decisions regarding the approval of new technology for coverage may vary from one local area to another (among other studies, see Foote et al. 2004), and small geographic variations may occur in the interpretation of the entitlement benefit package by intermediaries, carriers, and other entities that process claims.

4. As noted by the National Committee for Quality Assurance (2009), "HEDIS is a tool used by more than 90 percent of America's health plans to measure performance on important dimensions of care and service. . . . HEDIS consists of 71 measures across 8 domains of care. Because so many plans collect HEDIS data, and because the measures are so specifically defined, HEDIS makes it possible to compare the performance of health plans."

Chapter 2: Five Ways to Pay Medicare Health Plans

1. This section reflects MA payment policy through 2008 as a convenience to represent established policy through the Bush administration. Changes proposed or implemented by the Obama administration in 2009 are discussed separately below, as one of the five payment options.

2. U.S. Medicare Payment Advisory Commission 2008a, 254. This discussion omits certain complexities related to indirect medical education payments and "hold-harmless" provisions of risk adjustment in the calculation of the benchmark.

3. The average payment relative to FFS expenditures in large urban counties was 121 percent in 2006; in other floor counties, it was 134 percent (U.S. Medicare Payment Advisory Commission 2007b).

4. The growth in PFFS may come to an end in 2011, when PFFS plans will be required to develop formal provider networks in areas with at least two local network-based plans.

5. This paragraph could be interpreted as a suggestion that *all* beneficiaries have the choice of a private health plan, regardless of the cost required to induce private plan availability in all market areas—a suggestion that we reject later in this book.

6. It would be more accurate to say "on the margin" rather than "on average."

7. See introduction, above.

8. Some of the additional benefits beyond the entitlement probably were not efficient under the AAPCC, in the economic sense that they cost more than their value to beneficiaries (Dowd, Feldman, and Christianson 1996; Feldman et al. 2001). Given that MA plans now can offer premium rebates as well as other benefits, the current system and the MedPAC alternative provide benefits that are efficient.

9. Currently, these sources of benchmark pricing are the higher of urban and rural floors, a minimum annual update, a blended rate combining a local rate and the national average rate, and county-level per-capita FFS costs. Even the latter benchmark is more generous than the AAPCC, as the latter paid 95 percent of county-level FFS costs, not 100 percent.

10. The encounter data used in the HCC model are drawn from both FFS and HMO encounters.

11. See chapter 4 for our estimates of the savings from MedPAC's proposal and from competitive pricing.

12. He was indeed a major figure in the unsuccessful efforts of the HCFA (predecessor agency to the CMS) to establish an HMO-only competitive bidding demonstration in four cities in the late 1990s.

13. There is a strong argument for using competitive pricing to purchase equipment, supplies, and services for FFS Medicare, as well as for paying health plans. Our interest in this book is using competitive pricing to pay Medicare health plans, but we note these other uses.

14. This means that FFS, private fee-for-service (PFFS), and medical savings account (MSA) plans would have to participate in quality reporting.

15. Note that there is little reason in principle to assign medical education, disproportionate share, and other, similar costs solely to FFS. For example, MA plans have as much interest in a skilled workforce as do FFS providers. The bid adjustments suggested in the text take existing policy in these areas as given to keep the discussion focused on the five different payment options.

16. The Denver demonstration lacked one incentive that since has been offered to private plans that submit low bids—the opportunity to give premium rebates. This

additional incentive to private plans would have reduced the Denver bids by some additional, perhaps modest, amount.

17. Some MA plans have chosen to offer national service areas, but they are not required to do so.

18. Budget Director Peter Orszag has used the term "region" to describe the geographic unit for bidding (Carr 2009), but it is unclear whether he was speaking in generic terms—for example, region as something like a metropolitan statistical area—or he meant an area much larger than an MSA or the county unit currently used for bidding by local MA plans.

19. According to the U.S. Senate, Committee on Finance (2009, 40), the new benchmarks will be capped at the current MA benchmarks.

20. If bidding rules cap the benchmarks at FFS spending levels, then beneficiaries who prefer MA plans where FFS is cheaper will not impose an extra cost on the program.

Chapter 3: Technical Issues in Competitive Pricing for Medicare

1. At present, the weights are determined by the national FFS/MA enrollment percentages, respectively, so average plan bids for the region are assigned a weight of approximately one-fifth, while the average predetermined county rates are assigned a weight of four-fifths.

2. Thorpe and Atherly (2001) calculated private plans' costs in a way that avoided using ACR data. They started with 1997 data on the Medicare AAPCC and assumed that M+C plans could provide basic Medicare services for 80 percent of that cost. Then they trended this amount forward to 2002 at 5 percent per year. They estimated that private plans were 84 percent as costly as FFS in 2002. Finally, they assumed that private plans' bids would approximate plans' costs of providing basic Medicare services in 2002.

3. The submitted bid is always "just right" from an *a priori* perspective, but when other plans' bids are revealed, it may turn out to be too high if the other bids are lower than expected, or too low if the other bids are higher than expected.

4. In 2006, the regional benchmark was equal to 86 percent of the statutory component that was known in advance and 14 percent of the unknown plan bid component. Thus, it was neither a pure known nor unknown benchmark. Plans apparently responded, however, to the known component.

5. Rising marginal costs (MC) would be consistent with economies of scale if MC were less than average cost (AC). But it is unlikely that this condition would hold for long if MC were rising rapidly.

6. There is evidence that health plans have submitted unrealistic "low-ball" bids in the commercial health insurance market (Sutton, Feldman, and Dowd 2004).

Chapter 4: Estimating the Savings
from Competitive Pricing in Medicare

1. In particular, plans' bids might differ from their bids under the current payment system (a concern we discussed in chapter 3); beneficiaries could be more sensitive to price differences under competitive bidding (also discussed above); and differences in plans' bids might arise from differences in beneficiaries' health status that are not captured by the risk-adjustment mechanism (U.S. Congressional Budget Office 2006).

2. A reviewer asked why the numbers in table 4-3 are so much larger than the savings to Medicare in table 4-2. The numbers in table 4-3 are not enrollment-weighted because they show what a beneficiary in each cell would pay under each bidding model. For example, an MA enrollee living in an area of low FFS cost would pay $129.26 more per month (that is, average MA payment minus average FFS cost equals $129.26), but Medicare would save only $15.34 PMPM in the lowest-cost counties (calculation not shown).

3. Note that, if bidding rules cap benchmarks at FFS levels, these beneficiaries would be unaffected—there would be no premium rebate, because the benchmarks could not exceed FFS levels.

Chapter 5: Should FFS Medicare Be Allowed Greater Flexibility?

1. The same is true of entitlement benefits, but Congress has determined that the entitlement benefits must be offered, even if some beneficiaries do not value them at their cost.

2. That discussion has a precedent in Medicare because some MA plans have expressed interest in being able to demand FFS Medicare prices from their network providers.

3. On the opposition to negotiated drug prices, see Antos (2005), Frank (2004), and Frank and Newhouse (2008), among many other sources.

4. Private fee-for-service plans are exempt from these two requirements.

Chapter 6: The Uneasy Relationship of Competitive Bidding
to the Law and Politics of Medicare

1. U.S. Medicare Payment Advisory Commission 1999, 2003; Mutti 2003; Richard Beveridge and Associates 2001.

2. U.S. Medicare Payment Advisory Commission 1999; Coulam 1995.

3. Hoerger and Meadow 1997; Hoerger et al. 1998.

4. U.S. House of Representatives, Committee on Small Businesses 2007; Apolskis 2008; Reuters 2008; *Sharp v. Leavitt*, 2008 U.S. Dist. LEXIS 28623 (S.D. Cal.). See also §145 of the Medicare Improvements for Patients and Providers Act of 2008,

which withdraws authority from the CMS to conduct competitive bidding for clinical laboratory services (unlike Sec. 154 of that act, which *postpones* DME competitive bidding).

5. Coulam et al. 1990.

6. U.S. Department of Health and Human Services 2004; Karon et al. 2002.

7. Dowd et al. 2000; Karon et al. 2002; and *Florida Association of Medical Equipment Dealers v. Apfel*, 194 F. 3d 1227 (11th Cir. 1999).

8. *American Association of Homecare v. Leavitt*, 2008 U.S. Dist. LEXIS 49497 (D.D.C., 2008); *Carolina Medical Sales v. Leavitt*, 559 F. Supp. 2d 69 (D.D.C., 2008).

9. Section 154 of the Medicare Improvements for Patients and Providers Act of 2008.

10. Wayne 2008; Young 2008.

11 *American Association of Health Plans, Inc. v. Shalala*, Civil Action No. 97-WM-977 (D. Colo. May 12, 1997); Barnes 2005.

12. Dowd et al. 2000.

13. Ibid.

14. U.S. Department of Health and Human Services, Centers for Medicare and Medicaid Services 2008.

15. There are two types of private Part D plans: prescription drug plans (PDPs) and Medicare Advantage Prescription Drug plans (MA-PDs). Both submit annual bids, in the manner described in the text.

16. For a description of how plan bids translate into government payments and enrollee premiums, see MedPAC 2008c.

17. See discussions of the Part D bidding system in Antos (2005), Families USA (2007a), Frank (2004), Frank and Newhouse (2008), and Sipkoff (2007).

18. It is worth pointing out the obvious: Administrative pricing systems create losers as well as winners, in the form of providers who are penalized by the failure of administrative systems reliably to track the underlying costs of providing the services. Such losers have not been politically decisive in arguing for competitive pricing in past demonstrations.

19. At almost the same time, judges were denying efforts by the DME industry to stop the first phase of the nationwide DME competitive bidding program. In these cases, plaintiffs' claims focused on harms to DME suppliers, not to beneficiaries. See *American Association of Homecare v. Leavitt*, 2008 U.S. Dist. LEXIS 49497 (D.D.C., 2008); and *Carolina Medical Sales v. Leavitt*, 559 F. Supp. 2d 69 (D.D.C., 2008).

20. The main exceptions to this claim are the rural and urban floor payments which MedPAC and others now are challenging.

21. A temporary restraining order (TRO) is an emergency court order to prevent irreparable harm, or to maintain the status quo. As suggested by the name, a temporary restraining order is temporary. Ordinarily, before the TRO expires, an abbreviated adversarial hearing on a preliminary injunction must be scheduled (see, for example, Perlmutter 2007).

22. Two of the authors were present at the meeting.

23. For example, in the nationwide rollout of DME competitive bidding, excluded suppliers were able to make effective political appeals to Congress, protesting their exclusion.

24. Note our estimates in chapter 4, showing much lower savings from average-bid models of competitive pricing.

25. The exclusion of higher-cost suppliers creates an incentive for bidders to bid low without introducing added out-of-pocket costs for beneficiaries, as in the HMO bidding models.

26. HCPCS is a system of alphanumeric codes assigned to medical and surgical procedures, medications, supplies, equipment, and other components of health-care services and used for pricing and billing purposes. The HCPCS National Panel, a group composed of the CMS and other insurers, maintains the HCPCS codes.

Chapter 7: No Need for a Demonstration—
A Gradual Transition to Reform Should Start Now

1. MedPAC's finding, if generalizable to all newly entering plans, is a ringing indictment of higher payments to MA plans. Apparently, the new entrants are not able to offer the same quality as existing plans even when paid more; instead, they offer lower quality.

2. For example, Buchmueller (2000) estimated that a $10 increase (in 2008 prices) in the monthly FFS premium would reduce the FFS market share by 0.88 percentage points.

3. In two sites (Phoenix and Kansas City), the demonstrations were blocked after being mandated by Congress. The similarities to the 2010 CCA demonstration are striking and suggest a dysfunctional political decision-making process that bodes ill for the current level of direct congressional management of the Medicare program.

4. One example: Section 903 of HR 3162, a bill to reauthorize the Children's Health and Medicare Protection Act that passed the U.S. House of Representatives in 2007, contained a provision to repeal the 2010 demonstration.

5. For example, the CCA demonstration envisioned in the MMA would limit the change in out-of-pocket premiums that FFS enrollees could be required to pay to 5 percent per year, though we don't see any reason why such protection should be given to FFS enrollees only.

References

Abelson, R. 2008. Medicare Finds How Hard It Is to Save Money. *New York Times.* April 7.

Antos, Joseph R. 1991. The Policy Context of Physician Payment. In *Regulating Doctors' Fees: Competition, Benefits, and Controls Under Medicare*, ed. H. E. Frech III. Washington, D.C.: AEI Press.

———. 2005. Ensuring Access to Affordable Drug Coverage in Medicare. *Health Care Financing Review* 27 (2): 103–12.

Apolskis, Michael. 2008. U.S. District Court Stops Clinical Laboratory Competitive Bidding Demonstration. *Medicare Update.* April 12. http://medicareupdate. typepad.com/medicare_update/2008/04/on-april-8-2008.html (accessed August 3, 2009).

Areeda, Phillip, and Donald F. Turner. 1975. Predatory Pricing and Related Practices under Section 2 of the Sherman Act. *Harvard Law Review* 88 (4): 697–733.

Atherly, Adam. 2002. The Effect of Medicare Supplemental Insurance on Medicare Expenditures. *International Journal of Health Care Finance and Economics* 2 (2): 137–62.

Atherly, Adam, Bryan E. Dowd, and Roger Feldman. 2004. The Effect of Benefits, Premiums and Health Risk on Health Plan Choice in the Medicare Program. *Health Services Research* 39 (4, pt. 1): 847–64.

Balanced Budget Act of 1997, Public Law 33, 105th Cong., 1st sess. (August 5, 1997), Title IV.

Barnes, Julie. 2005. *Managed Care Litigation.* Washington, D.C.: Bureau of National Affairs.

Berenson, Robert A. 2004. Medicare Disadvantaged and the Search for the Elusive "Level Playing Field." *Health Affairs* Web Exclusive. December 15, w4-572–85. http://content.healthaffairs.org/cgi/reprint/hlthaff.w4.572v1 (accessed July 20, 2009).

———. 2008. From Politics to Policy: A New Payment Approach In Medicare Advantage. *Health Affairs* Web Exclusive, March 4, w156–64. http://content. healthaffairs.org/cgi/content/abstract/hlthaff.27.2.w156 (accessed July 20, 2009).

Berenson, Robert A., and Bryan Dowd. 2008. Medicare Advantage Plans at a Crossroads— Yet Again. *Health Affairs*, November 24, w29–40. ttp://content.healthaffairs.org/cgi/ content/abstract/28/1/w29 (accessed July 20, 2009).

Blumberg, Linda J., and Alison Evans. 1998. Reform of the Medicare AAPCC: Learn-
ing from Previous Proposals. *Inquiry* 35 (1): 62–77.

Booske, Bridget C., Judith Lynch, and Gerald Riley. 2002. Impact of Medicare Managed Care Market Withdrawal on Beneficiaries. *Health Care Financing Review* 24
(1): 95–115.

Borges, Bernhard F. J., and Jack L. Knetsch. 1997. Valuation of Gains and Losses, Fair-
ness and Negotiation Outcomes. *International Journal of Social Economics* 24
(1/2/3): 265–81.

Brown, Randall S., Dolores Gurnick Clement, Jerrold W. Hill, Sheldon M. Retchin,
and Jeanette W. Bergeron. 1993. Do Health Maintenance Organizations Work for
Medicare? *Health Care Financing Review* 15 (1): 7–23.

Buchmueller, Thomas C. 2000. The Health Plan Choices of Retirees Under Managed
Competition. *Health Services Research* 35 (5, pt. 1): 949–76.

Carr, Sean P. 2009. White House Official Outlines Medicare Advantage Bidding Plan.
A. M. Best via COMTEX. March 10. http://www3.ambest.com/frames/frameserver.
asp?site=news&tab=1&AltSrc=14&refnum=124444 (accessed August 28, 2009).

Cawley, John H., and Andrew B. Whitford. 2007. Improving the Design of Competitive Bidding in Medicare Advantage. *Journal of Health Politics, Policy and Law* 32
(2): 317–47.

Chiles, Lawton (governor of Florida). 1998. Letter to Nancy-Ann Min DeParle
(administrator of the Health Care Financing Administration). May 22.

Christensen, Sandra, Stephen H. Long, and Jack Rodgers. 1987. Acute Health Care
Costs for the Aged Medicare Population: Overview and Policy Options. *Milbank
Quarterly* 65 (3): 397–425.

Christianson, Jon B. 1987. Competitive Bidding for Home Care under the Channel-
ing Demonstration. *Health Care Financing Review* 8 (4): 73–86.

Cooper, Barbara, and Bruce C. Vladeck. 2000. Bringing Competitive Pricing to Medicare. *Health Affairs* 19 (5): 49–56.

Coulam, Robert. 1995. Contracting for Health Care Services: The Administrative
Problem. Unpublished paper. Abt Associates, Cambridge, Mass.

Coulam, Robert, and Gary Gaumer. 1991. Medicare's Prospective Payment System: A
Critical Appraisal. *Health Care Financing Review*, 1991 annual supplement, 45–77.

Coulam, Robert, Kevin Quinn, Leo Reardon, Alan White, Robert Schmitz, Nancy
Burstein, August Baker, and Carolyn Robinson. 1997. *Evaluation of the Effectiveness of the Operation Restore Trust Demonstration: Final Report*. Report submitted to
the Health Care Financing Administration pursuant to contract no. 500-92-
0014. September 29.

Coulam, Robert, and Leo Reardon. 1990. *Review of Reimbursement Methods of Other Pay-
ors for Durable Medical Equipment*. Report submitted by Abt Associates to the Health
Care Financing Administration pursuant to contract no. 500-85-0050. December 24.

Coulam, Robert, Leo Reardon, William Marder, Kathleen Calore, and Daniel Reck.
1990. *Final Report: Options for Medicare Reimbursement of Durable Medical*

Equipment. Report submitted by Abt Associates to the Health Care Financing Administration pursuant to contract no. 500-85-0050. December 24.

Davis, Steve. 2009. President Obama Targets $177 Billion in Medicare Advantage Rate Reductions to Help Fund Health Reform. *Health Plan Week.* March 11. http://www.aishealth.com/Bnow/hbd031109.html (accessed August 3, 2009).

Dixit, Avinash, and Susan Skeath. 2004. *Games of Strategy.* 2d ed. New York: W. W. Norton.

Dowd, Bryan. 2001. More on Competitive Pricing. *Health Affairs* 20 (1): 306–7.

Dowd, Bryan, Robert Coulam, and Roger Feldman. 2000. A Tale of Four Cities: Medicare Reform and Competitive Pricing. *Health Affairs* 19 (5): 9–29.

Dowd, Bryan, Robert Coulam, Roger Feldman, and Steven D. Pizer. 2005–6. Fee-for-Service Medicare in a Competitive Market Environment. *Health Care Financing Review* 27 (2): 113–26.

Dowd, Bryan, and Roger Feldman. 2002. Having It All: National Benefit Equity and Local Payment Parity in the Medicare Program. *Health Affairs* 21 (3): 208–14.

Dowd, Bryan, Roger Feldman, and Jon Christianson. 1996. *Competitive Pricing for Medicare.* Washington, D.C.: AEI Press.

Dowd, Bryan, Roger Feldman, and Robert Coulam. 2003. The Effect of Health Plan Characteristics on Medicare+Choice Enrollment. *Health Services Research* 38 (1, pt. 1): 113–35.

Duhigg, Charles. 2007. Golden Opportunities: Oxygen Suppliers Fight to Keep a Medicare Boon. *New York Times.* November 30.

Families USA. 2007a. Medicare Drug Plans Deliver Higher Prices. Publication No. 07-101. January. http://www.familiesusa.org/assets/pdfs/no-bargain-medicare-drug.pdf (accessed July 21, 2009).

———. 2007b. Whose Advantage? Billions in Windfall Payments Go to Private Medicare Plans. Publication No. 07-105. June. http://www.familiesusa.org/assets/pdfs/medicare-private-plans.pdf (accessed July 21, 2009).

Feldman, Roger, Bryan E. Dowd, Robert Coulam, Len Nichols, and Anne Mutti. 2001. Premium Rebates and the Quiet Consensus on Market Reform for Medicare. *Health Care Financing Review* 23 (2): 19–33.

Foote, Susan Bartlett, Douglas Wholey, Todd Rockwood, and Rachel Halpern. 2004. Resolving the Tug-Of-War Between Medicare's National and Local Coverage. *Health Affairs* 23 (4): 108–23.

Frank, Richard. 2004. Perspective: Election 2004—Prescription-Drug Prices. *New England Journal of Medicine* 351 (14): 1375–77.

Frank, Richard G., and Joseph P. Newhouse. 2008. Should Drug Prices Be Negotiated under Part D of Medicare? And If So, How? *Health Affairs* 27 (1): 33–43.

Freudenheim, Milt. 2003. Medicare Plan for Competition Faces Hurdles. *New York Times.* November 28.

Fuhrmans, Vanessa. 2009. Cuts Await Medicare Insurers. *Wall Street Journal.* February 26. http://online.wsj.com/article/SB123560916922977285.html (accessed July 21, 2009).

Fuhrmans, Vanessa, and Jane Zhang. 2009. U.S. Reduces Subsidies for Private Medicare. *Wall Street Journal*. April 7.

Given, Ruth S. 1996. Economies of Scale and Scope as an Explanation of Merger and Output Diversification Activities in the Health Maintenance Organization Industry. *Journal of Health Economics* 15 (6): 685–713.

Graham, Bob (U.S. Senator, D-FL). 1998. Graham Medicare Legislation Takes Root in Polk County. Press release. May 29.

Halpern, Rachel. 2005. M+C County Exit Decisions 1999–2001: Implications for Payment Policy. *Health Care Financing Review* 26 (3): 105–23.

Hanemann, W. Michael. 1991. Willingness to Pay and Willingness to Accept: How Much Can They Differ? *American Economic Review* 81 (3): 635–47.

Hoerger, Thomas, and Ann Meadow. 1997. Developing Medicare Competitive Bidding: A Study of Clinical Laboratories. *Health Care Financing Review* 19 (1): 59–86.

Hoerger, Thomas, Richard Lindrooth, and Jennifer Eggleston. 1998. Medicare's Demonstration of Competitive Bidding for Clinical Laboratory Services: What It Means for Clinical Laboratories. *Clinical Chemistry* 44 (8): 1728–34.

Hoffman, Elizabeth, and Matthew L. Spitzer. 1993. Willingness to Pay vs. Willingness to Accept: Legal and Economic Implications. *Washington University Law Quarterly* 71 (1): 59–114.

Horowitz, John H., and K. E. McConnell. 2003. Willingness to Accept, Willingness to Pay, and the Income Effect. *Journal of Economic Behavior and Organization* 51: 537–45.

Jencks, Stephen F., Timothy Cuerdon, Dale R. Burwen, Barbara Fleming, Peter M. Houck, Annette E. Kussmaul, David S. Nilasena, Diana L. Ordin, and David R. Arday. 2000. Quality of Care Delivered to Medicare Beneficiaries: A Profile at State and National Levels. *JAMA* 284 (13): 1670–76.

Kaiser Family Foundation. 2008. Fact Sheet: Medicare Advantage. September. http://www.kff.org/medicare/upload/2052-11.pdf (accessed July 21, 2009).

———. 2009. *Medicare: A Primer*. January. http://kff.org/medicare/upload/7615-02.pdf (accessed July 21, 2009).

KaiserNetwork.org. 2008. Daily Reports—Capitol Hill Watch: Lawmakers, Officials Discuss Overhauling U.S. Health Care System in 2009 during Senate Finance Committee Symposium. *Kaiser Daily Health Policy Report*. June 17. http://www.kaisernetwork.org/daily_reports/rep_index.cfm?DR_ID=52784 (accessed July 21, 2009).

Karon, Sara, Kay Jewell, Thomas Hoerger, Shulamit Bernard, Eric Finkelstein, Kevin Tate, Richard Lindrooth, and Teresa Waters. 2002. Evaluation of Medicare's Competitive Bidding Demonstration for DMEPOS: Second-Year Annual Evaluation Report. CMS Contract No. 500-95-0061/T.O. #3. April. www.cms.hhs.gov/DemoProjectsEvalRpts/downloads/2rtc_Appendix.pdf (accessed August 3, 2009).

Klevorick, Alvin K. 1993. The Current State of the Law and Economics of Predatory Pricing. *American Economic Review* 83 (2): 162–67.

Leland, Hayne E. 1972. Theory of the Firm Facing Uncertain Demand. *American Economic Review* 62 (3): 278–91.

Levit, Katharine, Cathy Cowan, Helen Lazenby, Arthur Sensenig, Patricia McDonnell, Jean Stiller, Anne Martin, and the Health Accounts Team. 2000. Health Spending in 1998: Signals of Change. *Health Affairs* 19 (1): 125–32.

Mathews, Anna Wilde. 2008. Lawmakers Question Medicare Bidding Plan. *Wall Street Journal* (eastern edition). May 6, A4.

Mathews, Merrill. 2006. Medicare's Hidden Administrative Costs: A Comparison of Medicare and the Private Sector. Council for Affordable Health Insurance. January 10. http://www.cahi.org/cahi_contents/resources/pdf/CAHI_Medicare_Admin_Final_Publication.pdf (accessed July 21, 2009).

Mayes, Rick, and Robert A. Berenson. 2006. *Medicare Prospective Payment and the Shaping of U.S. Health Care*. Baltimore, Md.: Johns Hopkins University Press.

McBride, Timothy D. 1998. Disparities in the Access to Medicare Managed Care Plans and Their Benefits. *Health Affairs* 17 (6): 170–80.

Medicare Improvements for Patients and Providers Act of 2008, Public Law 275, 110th Cong., 2d sess. (July 15, 2008), §145.

Medicare, Medicaid and SCHIP Balanced Budget Refinement Act of 1999 (BBRA), H.R. 3426, enacted by *Consolidated Appropriations Act of 2000*, Public Law 113, 106th Cong., 1st sess. (November 29, 1999), Division B.

Medicare, Medicaid, and SCHIP Benefits Improvement and Protection Act of 2000 (BIPA), H.R. 5661, incorporated in *Consolidated Appropriations Act of 2001*, Public Law 554, 106th Cong., 2d sess. (December 21, 2000), §1.

Medicare Prescription Drug, Improvement, and Modernization Act (MMA), Public Law 173, 108th Cong., 1st sess. (December 8, 2003), Title I.

Miller, Mark. 2008. Medicare Advantage Private Fee-for-Service Plans and Employer Groups. Presentation to National Health Policy Forum. April 11. http://nhpf.ags.com/handouts/Miller.slides_04-11-08.pdf (accessed August 3, 2009).

Miller, R. H., and H. S. Luft. 1997. Does Managed Care Lead to Better or Worse Quality of Care? *Health Affairs* 16 (5): 7–25.

———. 2002. HMO Plan Performance Update: An Analysis of the Literature, 1997–2001. *Health Affairs* 21 (4): 63–86.

Mutti, Ann. 2003. Experience with Market Competition in Fee-for-Service Medicare. Statement before a meeting of the Medicare Payment Advisory Commission. March 23. http://www.medpac.gov/transcripts/0321_feeforservice_AM_transc.pdf (accessed August 28, 2009).

National Committee for Quality Assurance. 2009. What is HEDIS? http://www.ncqa.org/tabid/187/Default.aspx (accessed September 11, 2009).

National Health Policy Forum. 2005. The Basics: Medicare Advantage. November 29. http://www.nhpf.org/pdfs_basics/Basics_MA_11-29-05.pdf (accessed October 22, 2008).

Newhouse, Joseph P., Melinda Beeuwkes Buntin, and John D. Chapman. 1997. Risk Adjustment and Medicare: Taking a Closer Look. *Health Affairs* 16 (5): 26–43.

Nichols, L. M., and R. D. Reischauer. 2000. Who Really Wants Price Competition in Medicare Managed Care? *Health Affairs* 19 (5): 30–43.

Obama, Barack. 2009. Remarks by the President at the Business Roundtable, St. Regis Hotel, Washington, D.C., March 12. Press release. www.whitehouse.gov/the_press_office/Remarks-by-the-President-at-the-Business-Roundtable (accessed August 3, 2009).

Omnibus Budget Reconciliation Act of 1989 (OBRA), Public Law 239, 101st Cong., 1st sess. (December 19, 1989), §1848.

Orszag, Peter. 2009. Remarks at 2009 Health Policy Forum, sponsored by America's Health Insurance Plans. March 10. Forum described at http://www.ahip.org/links/policy2009.

Parente, Stephen T., William N. Evans, Julie Schoenman, and Michael D. Finch. 2005. Health Care Use and Expenditures of Medicare HMO Disenrollees. *Health Care Financing Review* 26 (3): 31–43.

Perlmutter, Richard M. 2007. Interim Measures and Civil Litigation: Introduction. *Suffolk Transnational Law Review* 31 (1): 1–12.

Pizer, Steven D., Austin B. Frakt, and Roger Feldman. 2007. *Regional PPOs in Medicare: What are the Prospects?* Changes in Health Care Financing and Organizations. February. http://www.hcfo.net/pdf/ppo.pdf (accessed July 21, 2009).

Plott, Charles R., and Kathryn Zeiler. 2003. The Willingness to Pay/Willingness to Accept Gap, the Endowment Effect, Subject Misconceptions and Experimental Procedures for Eliciting Valuations. *American Economic Review* 95 (3): 530–45.

Pope, Gregory C., John Kautter, Randall Ellis, Arlene Ash, John Ayanian, Lisa Iezzoni, Melvin Ingber, Jesse Levy, and John Robst. 2004. Risk Adjustment of Medicare Capitation Payments Using the CMS-HCC Model. *Health Care Financing Review* 25 (4): 119–41.

Reichard, John. 2008. Obama Picking Early Fight with the Insurance Industry? *Commonwealth Fund Washington Health Policy Week in Review*. December 15. www.commonwealthfund.org/Content/Newsletters/Washington-Health-Policy-in-Review/2008/Dec/Washington-Health-Policy-Week-in-Review—December-15—2008/Obama-Picking-Early-Fight-with-the-Insurance-Industry.aspx (accessed July 21, 2009).

Reuters. 2008. Court Issues an Injunction in San Diego Clinical Laboratory Bidding Case. April 8. http://www.reuters.com/article/pressRelease/idUS13811+09-Apr-2008+BW20080409 (accessed July 21, 2009).

Richard Beveridge and Associates. 2001. Medicare Participating Centers of Excellence Demonstration for Cardiovascular Health Care Facilities Expanding in 2001. Unpublished paper.

Schmid, S. G. 1995. Geographic Variation in Medical Costs: Evidence from HMOs. *Health Affairs* 14 (1): 271–75.

Schoenman, Julie A., Stephen T. Parente, Jacob J. Feldman, Mona M. Shah, William N. Evans, and Michael D. Finch. 2005. Impact of HMO Withdrawals on Vulnerable Medicare Beneficiaries. *Health Care Financing Review* 26 (3): 5–30.

Sipkoff, Martin. 2007. What's Good for the VHA Is Not So Good for Medicare. *Managed Care*. February.

Skinner, Jonathan S., and Elliot Fisher. 1997. Regional Disparities in Medicare Expenditures: Opportunity for Reform. *National Tax Journal* 50 (3): 413–25.

Social Security Amendments of 1972, Public Law 603, 92d Cong., 2d sess. (October 30, 1972), §226.

Stigler, George J. 1947. The Kinky Oligopoly Demand Curve and Rigid Prices. *Journal of Political Economy* 55: 432–49.

Sutton, Harry, Roger Feldman, and Bryan Dowd. 2004. Disruption of a Managed Competition Environment by Low-Ball Premium Bids: The Minnesota State Employees Group Insurance Program. *North American Actuarial Journal* 8 (2): 73–83.

Tax Equity and Fiscal Responsibility Act of 1982 (TEFRA), Public Law 248, 97th Cong., 2d sess (September 3, 1982), §114.

Thorpe, Kenneth E., and Adam Atherly. 2001. Reforming Medicare: Impacts on Federal Spending and Choice of Health Plans. *Health Affairs* Web Exclusive. October 10, w51–64. http://content.healthaffairs.org/cgi/content/abstract/hlthaff.w1.51v1 (accessed July 21, 2009).

————. 2002. Medicare+Choice: Current Role and Near-Term Prospects. *Health Affairs* Web Exclusive. July 17, w242–52.

Town, Robert, and Su Liu. 2003. The Welfare Effect of Medicare HMOs. *Rand Journal of Economics* 34 (4): 719–36.

U.S. Boards of Trustees of the Federal Hospital Insurance and Federal Supplementary Medical Insurance Trust Funds. 2008. *2008 Annual Report*. March 25. http://www.cms.hhs.gov/ReportsTrustFunds/downloads/tr2008.pdf (accessed July 20, 2009).

————. 2009. *2009 Annual Report*. May 12. http://www.cms.hhs.gov/ReportsTrustFunds/downloads/tr2009.pdf.

U.S. Congressional Budget Office. 2006. *Designing a Premium Support System for Medicare*. December. http://www.cbo.gov/ftpdocs/76xx/doc7697/12-08-Medicare.pdf (accessed August 3, 2009).

U.S. Department of Health and Human Services. 2004. Final Report to Congress: Evaluation of Medicare's Competitive Bidding Demonstration For Durable Medical Equipment, Prosthetics, Orthotics, and Supplies. http://www.cms.hhs.gov/DemoProjectsEvalRpts/downloads/CMS_rtc.pdf (accessed August 3, 2009).

————. Centers for Medicare and Medicaid Services. 1999. Medicare Managed Care Contract Report. Data as of December 1 from monthly report summary MMCC-2003. http://www.cms.hhs.gov/HealthPlanRepFileData/04_Monthly.asp#TopOfPage (accessed August 3, 2009).

————. 2003. Medicare Managed Care Contract Report. Data as of December 1 from monthly report summary MMCC-2003. http://www.cms.hhs.gov/HealthPlanRep FileData/04_Monthly.asp#TopOfPage (accessed August 3, 2009).

————. 2007. Medicare Advantage in 2007. Updated April 20. http://www.cms.hhs. gov/MCRAdvPartDEnrolData/Downloads/MedicareAdvantageIn2007.zip (accessed August 28, 2009).

————. 2008. Competitive Acquisition for Part B Drugs and Biologicals: Overview. Updated through September 15. http://www.cms.hhs.gov/CompetitiveAcquisforBios (accessed August 3, 2009).

————. 2009. Issuance of the 2010 Call Letter. Letter from Jonathan Blum to Medicare Advantage Organizations and others. March 30. www.cms.hhs.gov/Prescription DrugCovContra/Downloads/2010CallLetter.pdf (accessed August 3, 2009).

————. n.d.a. Competitive Acquisition for DMEPOS. http://www.cms.hhs.gov/ DMEPOSCompetitiveBid/ (accessed August 28, 2009).

————. n.d.b. Medicare Enrollment: National Trends 1966–2008. Medicare Enrollment Reports. http://www.cms.hhs.gov/MedicareEnRpts/Downloads/HISMI08. pdf (accessed July 21, 2009).

U.S. Department of Health and Human Services. Competitive Pricing Advisory Committee. 1999. Design Report of the Competitive Pricing Advisory Committee. Report submitted to the Health Care Financing Administration. January 6. Copy available from coulam@simmons.edu.

————. 2001. Report to Congress. January 19. Copy available from coulam@ simmons.edu.

U.S. General Accounting Office. 1972. Need for Legislation to Authorize More Economical Ways of Providing Durable Medical Equipment Under Medicare: Report to the Congress by the Comptroller General of the United States. B-164031(4). May 12. http://archive.gao.gov/f0302/096573.pdf (accessed July 31, 2009).

————. 1997. Medicare HMOs: Setting Payment Rates Through Competitive Bidding. GAO/HEHS-97-154R. June 12. http://archive.gao.gov/paprpdf1/158828. pdf (accessed July 31, 2009).

U.S. Government Accountability Office. 2004. Past Experience Can Guide Future Competitive Bidding for Medical Equipment and Supplies. GAO-04-765. September. http://www.gao.gov/new.items/d04765.pdf (accessed August 3, 2009).

————. 2005. Report to the Committees on Armed Services, U.S. Senate and House of Representatives: Implementation Issues for New TRICARE Contracts and Regional Structure. GAO 05-773. July. http://www.gao.gov/new.items/d05773.pdf (accessed August 3, 2009).

————. 2008. Medicare: Competitive Bidding for Medical Equipment and Supplies Could Reduce Program Payments, But Adequate Oversight Is Critical. Highlights of GAO-08-767T, a testimony before the Subcommittee on Health, Committee on Ways and Means, House of Representatives. May 6. http://www.gao.gov/highlights/ d08767thigh.pdf (accessed August 3, 2009).

U.S. House of Representatives. Committee on Small Businesses. 2007. *Hearing on Competitive Bidding for Clinical Lab Services: Where It Is Heading and What Small Businesses Can Expect*. Medicare Clinical Lab Competitive Bidding Demo. 110th Cong., sess. 1. Statement of Timothy Love, director of ORDI, Centers for Medicare and Medicaid Services. July 25. Transcript in press release from CMS Office of Public Affairs. http://www.cms.hhs.gov/apps/media/press/testimony.asp? Counter=2370&intNumPerPage=10&checkDate=&checkKey=&srchType=1& numDays=3500&srchOpt=0&srchData=&keywordType=All&chkNews Type=7&intPage=&showAll=&pYear=&year=&desc=&cboOrder=date.

———. Committee on the Budget. 2007. *Medicare Advantage and the Federal Budget: A Hearing Before the Committee on the Budget*. 110th Cong., 1st sess. Testimony of Mark E. Miller, executive director, Medicare Payment Advisory Commission. June 28. http://frwebgate.access.gpo.gov/cgi-bin/getdoc.cgi?dbname=110_house_ hearings&docid=f:38252.pdf (accessed August 3, 2009).

U.S. Medicare Payment Advisory Commission. 1999. *Report to the Congress: Selected Medicare Issues*. June. http://www.medpac.gov/documents/Jun99%20Entire% 20report.pdf (accessed August 3, 2009).

———. 2003. *Report to the Congress: Variation and Innovation in Medicare*. June. http://www.medpac.gov/documents/June03_Entire_Report.pdf (accessed August 3, 2009).

———. 2004. *Report to the Congress: Medicare Payment Policy*. March. http:// www.medpac.gov/documents/Mar04_Entire_reportv3.pdf (accessed August 3, 2009).

———. 2007a. *Report to the Congress: Promoting Greater Efficiency in Medicare*. June. http://www.medpac.gov/documents/Jun07_EntireReport.pdf (accessed August 3, 2009).

———. 2007b. *Report to the Congress: Medicare Payment Policy*. March. http://www. medpac.gov/documents/030107_Testimony_Mar07_report.pdf (accessed August 3, 2009).

———. 2008a. *Report to the Congress: Medicare Payment Policy*. March. http://www. medpac.gov/documents/Mar08_EntireReport.pdf (accessed August 3, 2009).

———. 2008b. Medicare Advantage Program Payment System. *Payment Basics*. October. http://www.medpac.gov/documents/MedPAC_Payment_Basics_08_ MA.pdf (accessed August 3, 2009).

———. 2008c. "Part D Payment System: Payment Basics." Washington, D.C.: Med-PAC, revised October. http://www.medpac.gov/documents/MedPAC_Payment_ Basics_08_PartD.pdf (accessed August 3, 2009).

———. 2009. *Report to the Congress: Medicare Payment Policy*. March. http://www. medpac.gov/documents/Mar09_EntireReport.pdf (accessed August 3, 2009).

U.S. Office of Management and Budget. 2009. *Budget of the United States Government, Fiscal Year 2010*, February 26. http://www.whitehouse.gov/omb/budget (accessed August 3, 2009).

U.S. Senate. Committee on Finance. 2008. *Private Fee-for-Service Plans in Medicare Advantage: A Closer Look: A Hearing before the Committee on Finance.* 110th Cong., sess. 2. Testimony of Mark E. Miller, executive director of the U.S. Medicare Payment Advisory Commission. January 30. http://finance.senate.gov/hearings/testimony/2008test/013008mmtest.pdf (accessed June 30, 2009).

———. 2009. Description of Policy Options, Transforming the Health Care Delivery System: Proposals to Improve Patient Care and Reduce Health Care Costs. April 29. http://finance.senate.gov/sitepages/leg/LEG%202009/042809%20Health%20Care%20Description%20of%20Policy%20Option.pdf (accessed August 3, 2009).

Vickrey, William. 1961. Counterspeculation, Auctions, and Competitive Sealed Tenders. *Journal of Finance* 16 (1): 8–37.

Vistnes, Jessica P., Philip F. Cooper, and Gregory S. Vistnes. 2001. Employer Contribution Methods and Health Insurance Premiums: Does Managed Competition Work? *International Journal of Health Care Finance and Economics* 2 (1): 159–87.

Wayne, Alex. 2008. Once Bid, Twice Shy on Medicare Equipment Program. *Congressional Quarterly Weekly Online.* June 23, 1674–74. http://library.cqpress.com/cqweekly/weeklyreport110-000002902840 (accessed October 26, 2008).

Weinstein, Michael. 1999. Economic Scene: Rebates Could Smooth the Way for a Medicare Reform Plan. *New York Times.* September 23, C2.

Weissman, Joel S., Melissa Wachterman, and David Blumenthal. 2005. When Methods Meet Politics: How Risk Adjustment Became Part of Medicare Managed Care. *Journal of Health Politics, Policy and Law* 30 (3): 475–504.

Welch, W. P. 2002. Disease Management Practices in Health Plans. *American Journal of Managed Care* 8 (4): 353–61.

Whitford, Andrew. 2007. Designing Markets: Why Competitive Bidding and Auctions in Government Often Fail to Deliver. *Policy Studies Journal* 35 (1): 61–85.

Wholey, Douglas, Roger Feldman, Jon B. Christianson, and John Engberg. 1996. Scale and Scope Economies among Health Maintenance Organizations. *Journal of Health Economics* 15 (6): 657–84.

Williams II, Reginald D. 2005. Payment and Participation: A Renaissance for Medicare's Private Health Plans? Medicare Brief No. 12. National Academy of Social Insurance. May. http://www.nasi.org/usr_doc/medicare_brief_12.pdf (accessed August 3, 2009).

Young, Jeffrey. 2008. Business and Lobbying: Prescribing a Price Fix. *The Hill.* May 6. http://thehill.com/business—lobby/k-street-in-brief-2008-05-06.html (accessed July 21, 2009).

Index

About the Authors

Robert F. Coulam is a research professor and director of the Center for Health Policy Research at the Simmons School of Health Sciences. He was formerly a principal associate at Abt Associates, where he managed large-scale research and evaluation projects on Medicare and Medicaid policy issues. He has been active in research efforts supporting recent federal initiatives to reform the Medicare program. At Simmons, Dr. Coulam's primary responsibilities are to teach courses in health policy, law, and economics and to enhance the health program's research activities and funding. He also conducts research on the subjects of interrogation, terrorism, and international law. He received his PhD from the Kennedy School of Government and his JD from Harvard Law School.

Roger Feldman is the Blue Cross Professor of Health Insurance and a professor of economics in the Division of Health Policy and Management in the School of Public Health, University of Minnesota. Dr. Feldman was a Marshall Scholar at the London School of Economics and holds a PhD in economics from the University of Rochester. His research covers the organization, financing, and delivery of health care, with a focus on health insurance. He also studies competition among health-care providers and insurers. Currently, he is evaluating the effect of consumer-directed health plans on medical care costs and the use of preventive services. Dr. Feldman's experience in health-care policy includes serving on the senior staff of the President's Council of Economic Advisers, in which capacity he was the lead author of a chapter in the 1985 *Economic Report of the President*. From 1988 to 1992, he directed one of the four national research centers sponsored by the Centers for Medicare and Medicaid Services (CMS). In the 1990s, he advised the CMS on a demonstration of competitive pricing for

Medicare M+C plans and is currently evaluating Medicare's competitive pricing program for durable medical equipment. Dr. Feldman is a regular contributor to journals in economics and health services research. His research has received four "best paper" awards from the Association for Health Services Research and the National Institute of Health Care Management. He has been a consultant to the U.S. Department of Justice and several state agencies regarding health plan mergers and ownership changes.

Bryan E. Dowd is a professor in the Division of Health Policy and Management in the School of Public Health, University of Minnesota. His research focuses on health economics and health policy, including markets for public and private health insurance and health-care services, and the application of econometric methods to health service research problems. His recent research includes studies of insurance theory, causal modeling, health plan choice, enrollment and disenrollment in Medicare HMOs, tax policy, and Medicare reform. He received his PhD in public policy analysis from the University of Pennsylvania, his MS in urban administration from Georgia State University, and his BS in architecture from the Georgia Institute of Technology.

Jeremy A. Rabkin
Professor of Law
George Mason University
School of Law

Richard J. Zeckhauser
Frank Plumpton Ramsey Professor
of Political Economy
Kennedy School of Government
Harvard University

Research Staff

Gerard Alexander
Visiting Scholar

Ali Alfoneh
Visiting Research Fellow

Joseph Antos
Wilson H. Taylor Scholar in Health
Care and Retirement Policy

Leon Aron
Resident Scholar; Director of
Russian Studies

Paul S. Atkins
Visiting Scholar

Michael Auslin
Resident Scholar

Claude Barfield
Resident Scholar

Michael Barone
Resident Fellow

Roger Bate
Legatum Fellow in Global Prosperity

Walter Berns
Resident Scholar

Andrew G. Biggs
Resident Scholar

Edward Blum
Visiting Fellow

Dan Blumenthal
Resident Fellow

John R. Bolton
Senior Fellow

Karlyn Bowman
Senior Fellow

Alex Brill
Research Fellow

John E. Calfee
Resident Scholar

Charles W. Calomiris
Visiting Scholar

Lynne V. Cheney
Senior Fellow

Steven J. Davis
Visiting Scholar

Mauro De Lorenzo
Visiting Fellow

Christopher DeMuth
D. C. Searle Senior Fellow

Thomas Donnelly
Resident Fellow

Nicholas Eberstadt
Henry Wendt Scholar in Political
Economy

Jon Entine
Visiting Fellow

John C. Fortier
Research Fellow

David Frum
Resident Fellow

Newt Gingrich
Senior Fellow

Scott Gottlieb, M.D.
Resident Fellow

Kenneth P. Green
Resident Scholar

Michael S. Greve
John G. Searle Scholar

Kevin A. Hassett
Senior Fellow; Director,
Economic Policy Studies

Steven F. Hayward
F. K. Weyerhaeuser Fellow

Robert B. Helms
Resident Scholar

Frederick M. Hess
Resident Scholar; Director,
Education Policy Studies

Ayaan Hirsi Ali
Visiting Fellow

R. Glenn Hubbard
Visiting Scholar

Frederick W. Kagan
Resident Scholar

Leon R. Kass, M.D.
Hertog Fellow

Andrew P. Kelly
Research Fellow

Desmond Lachman
Resident Fellow

Lee Lane
Resident Fellow; Codirector,
AEI Geoengineering Project

Adam Lerrick
Visiting Scholar

Philip I. Levy
Resident Scholar

Lawrence B. Lindsey
Visiting Scholar

John H. Makin
Visiting Scholar

Aparna Mathur
Research Fellow

Lawrence M. Mead
Visiting Scholar

Allan H. Meltzer
Visiting Scholar

Thomas P. Miller
Resident Fellow

Charles Murray
W. H. Brady Scholar

Roger F. Noriega
Visiting Fellow

Michael Novak
George Frederick Jewett Scholar
in Religion, Philosophy, and
Public Policy

Norman J. Ornstein
Resident Scholar

Richard Perle
Resident Fellow

Ioana Petrescu
NRI Fellow

Tomas J. Philipson
Visiting Scholar

Alex J. Pollock
Resident Fellow

Vincent R. Reinhart
Resident Scholar

Michael Rubin
Resident Scholar

Sally Satel, M.D.
Resident Scholar

Gary J. Schmitt
Resident Scholar; Director of
Advanced Strategic Studies

Mark Schneider
Visiting Scholar

David Schoenbrod
Visiting Scholar

Nick Schulz
DeWitt Wallace Fellow; Editor-in-Chief,
American.com

Roger Scruton
Resident Scholar

Kent Smetters
Visiting Scholar

Christina Hoff Sommers
Resident Scholar; Director,
W. H. Brady Program

Tim Sullivan
Research Fellow

Phillip Swagel
Visiting Scholar

Samuel Thernstrom
Resident Fellow; Director,
AEI Press; Codirector, AEI
Geoengineering Project

Bill Thomas
Visiting Fellow

Alan D. Viard
Resident Scholar

Peter J. Wallison
Arthur F. Burns Fellow in
Financial Policy Studies

David A. Weisbach
Visiting Scholar

Paul Wolfowitz
Visiting Scholar

John Yoo
Visiting Scholar